NATURAL BEAUTY

Health and beauty are inseparable, and this book
shows the natural way to achieve both.

NATURAL BEAUTY

Radiant Good Looks the Healthy Way

by

CAROL HUNTER

NATURE'S WAY

THORSONS PUBLISHERS LIMITED
Wellingborough, Northamptonshire

First published 1979
Second Impression 1981
Third Impression 1983

ISBN 0 7225 0515 9

Printed and bound in Great Britain by
Richard Clay (The Chaucer Press) Ltd.,
Bungay, Suffolk

CONTENTS

CHAPTER ONE

WHAT IS NATURAL BEAUTY?

You could spend hundreds of pounds on trying to improve your looks with expensive cosmetics and beauty salon treatments, only to find, at the end of it all, that you looked little better than before you started. You might pass as a beauty from a distance, but anyone taking a closer look would be in for a shock. This is because the best such measures can achieve is to mask any imperfections or blemishes you may have – they can never give you those basic attributes which go to make up a natural beauty.

Natural beauty is a rare quality which has as much to do with clear skin, bright eyes and shining hair as it does with perfect features. And while you cannot change your features, you can work towards attaining these other basic requirements of natural beauty.

The trouble is that although most people are concerned about their looks, few are prepared to put in any effort when it comes to improving their appearance. Yet, as you will find when you read this book, many of the measures advocated for beauty will also benefit your health. And a basic beauty routine, once you get into the swing of it, will take up only a few minutes of your time each day.

The earlier you start to care for your looks the better, and if mothers were more fastidious about introducing their children to a beauty care routine, they might encounter fewer beauty problems during the teens. Don't give up hope, however, if this period of your life is little more than a hazy memory, for it is never too late to start beauty treatment. The results may be less spectacular, but you'll find that perseverance will pay off whatever your age.

GIVING NATURE A HELPING HAND

Some people feel that nature should be left to her own devices when it comes to their appearance, but there are ways in which you can improve your looks without compromising a belief in doing things the natural way. And, as you will see later, beauty is closely related to your health and diet, as well as to how much sleep, fresh air and exercise you get.

Certainly there is an element of vanity involved in caring for your looks, but an attractive appearance not only pleases the beholder. It also gives the person concerned an added feeling of confidence which is reflected in other areas of their life. You know yourself how much better you feel mentally when you know that you are looking your best.

Cosmetics can play their part in natural living too. The cosmetic business is a large and lucrative one, and the companies in this field make millions of pounds from pandering to the vanity of both men and women. Every year more weird and wonderful products emerge from the laboratory, packed full of chemicals, decked out in elaborate packaging, and complete with nebulous promises of eternal youth and longer-lasting beauty. It is ironic that many people carefully avoid refined processed foods in their diet, while blithely applying synthetic cosmetics to their body.

There are trends in beauty, as in most things, and recent years have seen a tremendous upsurge in the popularity of natural cosmetcis. These are made from herbs, plants and other natural ingredients, many of which have been used for hundreds of years for their beautifying properties. The manufacturers of these products try, as far as possible, to avoid the use of synthetic ingredients and chemical additives, believing that natural ingredients work in harmony with the body.

It is an idea with undoubted aesthetic appeal, but it's also a fact that natural cosmetics seldom produce rashes or allergic reactions in even the most sensitive of skins. The same cannot be said for the mass-produced cosmetics, which often contain a wealth of hidden chemical ingredients.

Until the contents of cosmetics have to be declared, there is no way of knowing just what goes into a particular product, but it pays to be careful since even the so-called 'natural' cosmetics on the mass market are usually synthetic products with herbal ingredients added. Their addition is used by the manufacturers as a good selling point, taking advantage of the current trend towards all things natural.

LOOK IN YOUR HEALTH FOOD SHOP
The best hunting ground for natural cosmetics is your health food shop. Here you will find a wide range of products, many of which have an interesting and appealing story behind them. Some may have been produced by hand in the maker's own kitchen, while others will have been made from herbs and plants freshly picked on the very day of manufacture.

Among the natural ingredients, you'll find such appetizing substances as cucumber, honey, fruit juices and vegetable oils. Herbs like rosemary, chamomile and lavender are popular ingredients, while essential oils (obtained by distilling flowers) are used to impart a delicate fragrance and to enliven the circulation.

The small companies in this market believe in letting their products speak for themselves. Most don't spend thousands of pounds on fancy packaging or extensive advertising (they couldn't afford to!), which means they can sell their cosmetics at prices which compare very favourably with those on the mass market.

The cosmetic industry is one of the worst offenders when it comes to cruelty to animals. The manufacture of cosmetics involves some barbaric tests on animals, which cannot fail to disgust even the hardest of hearts. Natural cosmetics are seldom subjected to such tests and have no need to be. Indeed many of the companies concerned have a vegetarian background, and so do not even include animal ingredients in their products.

You may notice an absence of make-up from the health food shop. This is not so much because the customers don't believe in it, as that these items are almost impossible to make without the inclusion of synthetic ingredients. While they may fulfil other criteria (e.g., vegetarianism), they are rarely completely natural.

NOT FORGETTING THE MEN

No beauty book would be complete without at least a mention of men and their looks. Gone are the days when men were considered effeminate if they so much as used a deodorant, and the proliferation of after shaves, hair lotions, and even make-up, designed with men in mind, suggests that the male population is at last admitting an interest in its appearance.

Most men, however, would still shudder at the thought of taking any steps to maintain or improve their looks. They might stop to think twice about it if they realized that such common male problems as dry skin, open pores, red veins, or dandruff could be eliminated if they took a little care of themselves. So, for those men who *are* convinced: the advice contained in this book is just as relevant as it is to women, and while no one expects you to 'go the whole hog', you could at least carry out the basic rudiments without compromising your dignity.

CHAPTER TWO

BEAUTY IS MORE THAN SKIN DEEP

To the trained eye, your skin, hair, eyes, nails and teeth all have a story to tell. The condition they are in gives a good indication both of your general state of health, and of any deficiencies in your diet. For instance, when somebody is under the weather their hair, skin and eyes quickly lose their natural lustre, and instead look dull and tired. In the same way, such common beauty problems as broken nails or falling hair can all too often be traced back to a deficiency in the diet (in these two cases, of the B vitamins).

Just as diet and health are closely related, so too are diet and beauty. And, as we have just seen, health also has a close bearing on beauty. What you eat (or don't eat) has a dramatic effect on your outward appearance as well as your physical well-being.

EATING FOR BEAUTY

What is the right sort of diet to choose for improved looks? Ideally it is one which supplies a sufficient quantity of all the nutrients essential both to health and beauty. At the end of this chapter you will find a chart listing the nutrients of particular importance to beauty, together with their main sources. As you will see from this list, when this is translated in terms of food it represents a diet based on wholefoods and incorporates plenty of fresh raw fruit and vegetables.

Wholefoods are those which are as near as possible to their natural state, and as such they contain the maximum amount of nutrients. These foods have not been subjected to rigorous refining processes which destroy many valuable nutrients, and where possible wholefoods are free from the artificial additives which are so widely used in refined foods. It is by choosing wholefoods, and avoiding the many processed foods on the market, that you can build up health and vitality through diet.

A wholefood diet would include the following:

WHOLEMEAL FLOUR

This contains 100 per cent of the original wheat grain, complete with vitamins E, B, A, protein, unsaturated fat and natural roughage. During the production of white flour many valuable nutrients are lost (including the wheat germ and bran, which are removed). Since only four of these nutrients are replaced by synthetic equivalents, the natural balance of the wheat grain is completely upset. Wholemeal flour is also free from additives of any description, unlike white flour which contains a long list of chemicals designed to improve its appearance, texture and keeping properties. Even wholemeal bread is allowed to contain a certain number of additives like emulsifiers, stabilizers and preservatives, so the answer is really to bake your own. You will find that with a little practice wholemeal flour can be used for all your baking requirements, and once you've adjusted to the new taste you'll also enjoy the improved flavour.

WHOLEGRAIN CEREALS

Just as wholemeal flour contains more goodness than white, so the wholegrain cereals are richer in nutrients than their refined equivalents. Wholegrains are rich in vitamins E and B (especially riboflavin, thiamine, niacin, pantothenic acid and B6), as well as being a good source of protein and natural roughage. Into this category come breakfast cereals, pasta, rice, and less well-known grains like rye, barley and buckwheat.

RAW SUGAR

No sugar is good for you, and since a high sugar

intake is linked with such diseases as diabetes and coronary thrombosis, you should cut down on sugar in any form. White sugar provides nothing but calories, although raw sugar contains small quantities of vitamins and minerals, in particular calcium, iron, phosphorus and the B vitamins. Since raw sugar is stronger in taste than white, you'll also find that you need to use less of it to achieve the same degree of sweetness. Other natural sweeteners to use in place of sugar are honey, molasses and dried fruit, all of which provide many valuable nutrients.

VEGETABLE FATS

A high intake of saturated fats, chiefly from animal sources, has been strongly linked with coronary and vascular diseases. The Royal College of Physicians has recommended people to cut their total fat intake by one third, and to switch to those fats which are unsaturated, i.e. vegetable fats. Coconut oil is one vegetable fat which is highly saturated (although it is widely used by food manufacturers), so when buying vegetable oil or margarine it is worth checking that it is in fact unsaturated. The oils highest in polyunsaturates are, in descending order, safflower, sunflower, corn, cotton seed, soya, wheat germ, sesame and peanut.

Anyone who is inclined to greasy skin or hair should take care to limit their fat intake, although fats should never be totally excluded from the diet since they are required to maintain healthy cells and skin structure. Conversely, those with dry skin or hair, should add a tablespoonful of vegetable oil to their daily diet, preferably in the form of salad dressing, since fried foods simply add unwanted calories and make foods less digestible.

FRUIT AND VEGETABLES

These are an excellent source of a wide range of vitamins, minerals and roughage, especially when eaten raw, since cooking destroys many nutrients. Eat as many of these foods as you can, making sure that you include at least one salad each day.

PROCEED WITH CAUTION

Having chosen the ingredients of your diet with care, you must then proceed to prepare and cook them carefully if you are to avoid unnecessary destruction of nutrients. Vitamins and minerals are extremely unstable substances, and can easily be destroyed by such common factors as storage, exposure to air, heat or water.

Foods should be cooked as and when they are required, rather than being left to soak or to stand around. Roast or grill foods rather than frying them, and cook at low temperatures for the shortest possible time. Always serve at once, rather than keeping hot or reheating.

Particular care should be taken with vegetables, which should not be peeled before cooking since many nutrients are contained in and immediately under the skin. Wash and chop vegetables immediately prior to cooking, and use the minimum amount of liquid: vegetables do not need to be immersed – $\frac{1}{2}$ pt. (275ml) of liquid is ample to cook vegetables for four people. Plunge vegetables straight into boiling water, and cook for the minimum length of time. When cooked, vegetables should retain some of their original crunchiness. Reserve the cooking liquid, which is by now rich in nutrients, for use in soups, casseroles or drinks.

PLANNING A MENU

A basic menu would be as follows:

Breakfast:
　　Freshly squeezed fruit juice
　　Muesli served with wheat germ, fresh fruit and
　　unsweetened yogurt
　　Wholemeal bread and honey
　　Milk or herb tea

Lunch:
  Mixed vegetable salad with a dressing of yogurt and
    lemon juice, or cider vinegar and vegetable oil
  Wholemeal bread and low fat cheese or lean meat
  Fresh fruit
  Fruit juice or herb tea

Supper:
  Home-made soup
  Egg or cheese dish, or meat or fish, served with
    lightly cooked vegetables
  Fresh fruit salad or a fruit-based dessert
  Decaffeinated coffee or herb tea

In addition to this you should drink plenty of liquids, in the form of five or six glasses of water or fruit juice daily.

VITAMINS FOR BEAUTY

As you will see from the chart, the vitamins each have a part to play in the way you look. **Vitamin A**, for instance, is essential for proper eyesight, especially at night time. Those who use their eyes a lot, such as typists or draughtsmen, need extra quantities of this vitamin. Problems with the eyes are often a sign of a vitamin A deficiency. A shortage of this vitamin can also cause the skin to become clogged, leading to blemishes and rough skin resembling gooseflesh, the latter being most common on the upper arms, the knees and thighs.

The Vitamin B Complex is involved in controlling skin secretions, and as such is vital for healthy skin and hair. The B vitamins also help counteract stress, which takes a heavy toll on our appearance. The best source of the complex is brewer's yeast, which not only contains the whole B complex, but has 14 minerals, 17 amino acids, and a high proportion of the protein needed for healthy hair and skin. Take it in tablet form, or add the powder to cereals, stews, baked dishes, etc.

Vitamin C helps to purify and revitalize the blood stream, and so is essential for good skin. Since this.

vitamin cannot be stored in the body, it is vital to obtain a daily intake.

Vitamin D's prime role is the part it plays in bone formation, together with the minerals calcium and phosphorus. It is also needed for healthy teeth, and a deficiency appears to be linked with dental decay.

Vitamin E is one of the latest discoveries in the beauty field, and has had many miraculous claims made for it. An increasing number of women swear by its ability to heal scar tissue, and to delay and diminish wrinkles. Vitamin E is applied externally for cosmetic purposes, but should also be eaten for a better complexion resulting from improved circulation. Wheat germ is one of the best sources, and it's also rich in protein and vitamin A.

OTHER IMPORTANT FACTORS

Diet is not the only factor with a direct effect on your looks. Almost as important is the need for adequate sleep, fresh air and exercise, all of these being vital for looks as well as for health. Proper elimination and correct posture also have an important part to play in the way you look.

SLEEP

Although individual requirements vary considerably, most people find that around eight hours sleep a night is the ideal amount. If you have difficulty in sleeping, try taking a warm drink, such as hot milk with honey or molasses, before going to bed. Avoid burning the candle at both ends, since this will not only make you feel tense and irritable, but will be reflected in dark bags and lines around the eyes.

FRESH AIR

Breathing is something we do automatically and unconsciously, but in fact it's a pity that people don't think more about their breathing. If they did they would find that their usual rate of breathing is shallow and does not make full use of the lungs.

Breathing should be deep, relaxed and regular – correct breathing stimulates the circulation by increasing the flow of oxygen around the body. Make sure your rooms are well-ventilated (including the bedroom), and try to get some fresh air every day. If you have central heating, use a humidifier or place a bowl of water near the heater to maintain the correct humidity.

ELIMINATION

Constipation gives skin a grey, tired look, dulls the eyes, and makes the hair lank and lifeless. If you are eating a wholefood diet you should have little trouble with constipation. However, if you do suffer at all, include two tablespoonsful of natural bran in your daily diet, by adding it to cereals, soups, stews, drinks, or using it in baking.

EXERCISE

Few people take enough exercise, and in fact most are lucky if they get any at all. Exercise not only improves the circulation, but helps to tone up the body by firming the muscles and giving flexibility. Ideally you should take some exercise daily, even if it is no more than a brisk walk. There is no point in going mad on exercise one day each week, only to relapse into your usual slothful habits for the rest of the week.

The most effective forms of exercise are swimming and jogging, since both of these employ almost every muscle in the body. For those who are not interested in the many sporting activities available, exercise can take the form of a set series of movements. There are many different forms, but they have one basic thing in common, and that is that they require a tremendous amount of willpower if they are to be practised regularly. This is why many people find group keep fit or exercise classes of value.

Here is a simple set of exercises with which you

ould start to get yourself in shape. Begin first thing in the morning, before you even get out of bed, by really stretching your body from head to toe. Then relax for a few minutes (without going back to sleep!). Repeat this exercise when you get up.

With the following exercises start off with a few minutes each day, gradually building up the length of time.

Arms
Stand upright, feet together, and swing your arms backwards and fowards as high and as hard as possible.

Bust
With your arms level with your shoulders, elbows out, press the palms of your hands together. Count to ten and then relax.

Stomach
This is one of the worst offenders as far as sagging muscles go. Lie on your back on the floor, hands by your side and legs out straight. Lift your legs slowly until they are at right angles to the ground. When your feet are six inches from the floor, hold this position for a count of six before continuing to lower them to the ground.

Waist
Stand with your feet apart, hands stretched above your head. Circle the top part of your body, trying to touch the floor and then reach up as high as you can. Don't bend your knees. Repeat, rotating the body in the other direction.

Back
Lie on your front, arms bent, and with your head resting on your hands. With your legs straight, lift one at a time as high up behind you as you can. Hold

and then slowly lower to the floor. Repeat with the other leg.

Bottom
Sit on the floor, arms and legs out straight in front of you. 'Walk' backwards and forwards on your bottom.

Legs
Stand with feet together, arms by your sides. Bend your knees while keeping your heels on the floor. Repeat three times, then raise your heels off the ground and bend right down as low as you can. Rise slowly, bringing hands up over your head with arms straight.

POSTURE
Many a potential beauty has been marred by poor posture. In fact this must be the most common of all beauty problems, although it is not often recognized as such. Standing, walking and sitting incorrectly not only spoil your looks, but put an unnecessary strain on the bones and joints which can result in backache and other postural complaints. Incorrect posture can also limit the supply of oxygen if the chest and lungs are cramped, and can be involved in digestive troubles. Good posture, on the other hand, helps to improve the figure.

The first step towards good posture is to learn how to stand correctly, and to conquer this it helps to position yourself in front of a full-length mirror. Stand up straight, and imagine a thread running up through your body and head which lifts and stretches the whole body. If you find this difficult to imagine, hang a piece of weighted string from the top of your mirror as a guide. Pull your stomach in, tuck your buttocks under, with chest high, and shoulders pulled back but relaxed. If it feels uncomfortable, this is a sure sign that your usual stance leaves much to be desired.

This is the posture you should maintain for walking too. Step out with your toes straight ahead, and your arms swinging in a relaxed way as you walk. Move from the thighs rather than the hips, remembering to keep your back straight. Hold your head straight too, with chin up, and breathe deeply. When you are sitting, try and sit upright – you'll find this easier on a hardbacked chair, than on one of the inviting, soft-cushioned, modern lounging chairs. Correct posture while sitting is particularly important for those with sedentary jobs. Check that your desk and chair are the correct height – your feet should rest flat on the floor, with your bottom right to the back of the chair, and your back straight.

It is impossible to break the habits of a lifetime overnight, and the only way you are likely to improve your posture is to take regular checks on the way you stand, walk and sit. Whenever it occurs to you, check to see what your faults are, and correct them as described above. You will find that it becomes easier with practice, so it is worth persevering.

ENEMIES OF BEAUTY

Other habits that are likely to have an adverse affect on your looks as well as your health are alcohol, smoking, and stress. **Alcohol** not only uses up the B vitamins which, as already mentioned, play an important part in beauty, but it also encourages the appearance of thread veins, which are almost impossible to eradicate. **Smoking** is said to encourage the formation of wrinkles, and although there is no scientific proof of this, it is a fact that each cigarette uses up 25mg of vitamin C. Since this is almost equivalent to the minimum recommended daily intake (which is 30mg), anyone who smokes heavily is almost certain to be short of this important nutrient.

Stress, of course is less under our control, especially in the high-pressured society in which most of us live. However, stress can be conquered to a large extent if the correct mental attitude is adopted. Many people find that the regular practice of yoga, meditation or relaxation techniques helps them to combat stress, and anybody who is subjected to undue stress in their daily life would be well advised to enquire about these. Otherwise, you will find that the signs of tension will be all too obvious, in a drawn appearance with early wrinkles – and not the laughter lines which can add character to a face, but the worried frown lines.

FOODS FOR BEAUTY

Nutrient and Main Function	Main Dietary Sources
VITAMIN A for healthy hair and eyes, resistance to infections (which can lead to acne), suntanning. Also counteracts dandruff, dry skins and wrinkle formation. Needed for healthy circulation.	Fish liver oils, liver and other offal, dairy produce, eggs, carrots, spinach, watercress, apricots.
VITAMIN B COMPLEX for healthy hair and skin. A deficiency can lead to oily hair, dandruff, dry skin, redness and irritations, wrinkles and poor hair growth.	Wholewheat bread and flour, wholegrains, liver, wheat germ, brown rice, molasses, meat, fish, brewer's yeast.
VITAMIN C for hair, eyes and teeth, resistance to infection, healing of wounds, firm skin tissues. Dry skin and thread veins can be caused by a deficiency.	Green vegetables, fresh fruit, especially citrus fruits, blackcurrants, rose hips, green peppers.
VITAMIN D for healthy teeth, bones and nails. Essential for the assimilation of calcium and phosphorus.	Fish liver oils, eggs, butter, margarine.
VITAMIN E to prevent wrinkles, dry skin, brown age spots and dandruff. Helps to improve circulation and healing of scars.	Wholewheat bread, wholegrains, wheat germ, eggs, nuts, vegetable oils.
PROTEIN for healthy hair, skin, teeth and nails. For firm skin tissues.	Meat, fish, dairy produce, nuts, pulses, wheat germ, brewer's yeast.
FATS to counteract dry skin and hair and for assimilation of fat soluble vitamins A, D, E, and K.	Butter, margarine, vegetable oils, nuts, egg yolk.
CALCIUM and PHOSPHORUS work together for healthy teeth, hair, nails and bones.	*Calcium:* eggs, dairy produce, green vegetables. *Phosphorus:* As calcium, plus nuts, wheat germ, meat, pulses.

CHAPTER THREE

ALL YOU NEED TO KNOW ABOUT SKIN CARE

Skin care is rather like health – it is something we tend to ignore until signs of neglect begin to show. It is only when a revealing glance in the mirror one day reveals wrinkles, spots or blemishes which never used to be there that, in a sudden panic, we resolve to pay more attention to our poor old face – by which time, of course, it takes extra care and effort to repair the damage, because with beauty (as with health) prevention is easier than cure.

Proper care of the skin is vital at any age. When you are young, it helps to prevent such common teenage problems as greasy skin and acne, while as you grow older it is important to counteract the increasing dryness of the skin. You can have a beautiful skin at any age if you know how to care for it.

When we talk about skin care we usually refer to the face because this area, more than any other, needs care and attention (we'll get round to the other areas later in the chapter). Your face is constantly exposed to the elements, even in the depths of winter when the rest of you is well-wrapped up. That iş why the face is one of the first parts to show signs of ageing.

GETTING TO KNOW YOUR SKIN

Although the skin is the most obvious part of the body, surprisingly few people are aware of its structure, or of the many important functions it performs. The skin forms a protective barrier against harmful bacteria and infections. At the same time, it is a means of eliminating waste matter from the body, in the form of excess water, toxins, and carbon dioxide. The skin also has a part to play as a sense organ, in regulating the body temperature, in respiration, and in the metabolic processes of the body.

The skin is divided into three layers, and it is from the innermost layer that the various glands, including the oil and sweat glands, penetrate to the surface to eliminate waste matter. This inner layer, which is based on the fatty adipose tissue of the lower dermis, also acts as a cushion for the rest of the skin. It contains the finely distributed muscles of the skin which are involved in regulating body temperature. It is when these muscles contract that gooseflesh is formed on the surface of the skin.

The most important function of the middle skin layer, known as the dermis, is respiration. It is here that the countless tiny blood vessels, or capillaries, end in finely drawn networks, from where they feed the upper layer of skin which contains no blood vessels. It is the dermis which determines skin tone.

The third, or outer layer of the skin is the epidermis, which ranges in thickness from 1/20th of an inch on the palms and soles, to 1/200th of an inch on the face. The epidermis consists of several layers of cells, the outer layers being constantly shed as new layers grow up to replace them. It is this skin layer which contains the nerve endings, and the oil and sweat glands also open in the epidermis.

FIRST THINGS FIRST
How, then, do you begin to care for this complex organ which is your skin? Before you can take any steps to improve your complexion, you must first decide what skin type you have. Although the same basic rules apply to all types, certain modifications need to be made, as you will see from the chart at the end of this chapter.

The simple way to identify your skin type if you do not instantly recognize it from the descriptions in the chart, is to position yourself in daylight with a mirror (a magnifying one if you feel brave enough).

Wash your face with warm water and a little mild soap, then pat dry. Take a tissue and press it to your face, concentrating on the area around the nose and the chin. If your skin is greasy there will be definite traces of oil on the tissue. A dry skin, on the other hand, will feel taut and stretched, while a normal skin will show little or no reaction. A combination skin is one which combines the characteristics of a greasy skin with those of a dry or normal one. Usually the centre panel of the face (i.e. the forehead, nose and chin) is inclined to be greasy since this area contains more sebaceous glands than any other area of the body. At the same time, the skin on the cheeks is dry. With a combination skin you should treat each area separately, as indicated in the chart.

Even though it is possible to divide skin into one of these four categories, you will find that your skin may react very differently to that of somebody else with apparently the same skin type. For this reason the choice of cosmetics is a very individual matter, and the only way to find a product that suits you is to try many different types. Use any new cosmetic for at least two weeks to allow your skin time to adjust to it. If you then find the product unsuitable, progress to another one, always choosing cosmetics designed specifically for your skin type.

ESTABLISHING A ROUTINE

If you really want to improve your complexion you must establish a daily routine over an indefinite period – unfortunately a beautiful skin does not materialize overnight! Talk of routine may sound tedious, especially if you've been getting away with soap and water for years without any untoward effect, but it is really a small price to pay for longer-lasting beauty.

There are three basic steps in a skin care programme, which should be repeated night and morning. Once you get into the habit, you will find that they take no more than a few minutes of your time.

CLEANSING

First and foremost, you must keep your skin thoroughly cleansed, for it is inadequate cleansing which is responsible for many skin problems. Don't be deceived if your skin *looks* clean – you'll be amazed at how much hidden dirt appears on the cotton wool when you use a good cleanser. Proper cleansing not only removes all the dust, dirt and make up which accumulate during the day. It also stops the oil-secreting sebaceous glands from getting clogged up, which can lead to spots and blackheads. This means that cleansing is especially important for greasy skins, to remove pore-clogging oil and dead cells.

The type of cleanser you choose will be governed by your skin type. A dry skin, for instance, will benefit from a creamy cleansing lotion, while a greasy skin is better with one of the rinseable cleansers. When applying a cleanser or any other lotion to the face and neck, always use an upward outward motion. This prevents the skin from being stretched in the wrong direction, and also stimulates the circulation of blood which nourishes the skin. The only exception to this rule is a toner, which should be gently patted on to the skin. Extra care should be taken when cleansing around the nostrils, since this is the oiliest part of the face. Include the eye area, but treat it with care since the skin here is very thin and delicate.

TONERS AND ASTRINGENTS

Having thoroughly cleansed your skin, now is the time to apply a toner or astringent. Since astringents have a higher alcohol content than toners (alcohol having a drying effect), these are more suited to greasy skins. However, even a greasy skin needs only a mild astringent, or flakiness may result. Both a toner and an astringent serve the same purpose, namely to remove the last traces of cleanser, to freshen the skin and close the pores.

Those who say their skin does not feel really clean unless they wash with water should try using a toner, which has a more invigorating effect. If you are still not convinced, settle for one of the deep-acting, liquid cleansers which are washed rather than wiped off. If you're using water, it should always be tepid, since extremes of temperature could encourage the formation of thread veins. When you have washed and patted dry your face, apply a toner as described above.

MOISTURISERS

Last but not least comes the moisturiser, and it is this which helps the skin retain its youthful look, by forming a film to offset unwanted evaporation of water. A moisturiser gives moisture to the skin cells, thus lubricating and softening them. Whether your skin is dry or greasy, it still needs regular moisturising, and this is a habit to acquire early in life, since the skin begins to lose its natural moisture and elasticity as early as twenty years old. During the day a moisturiser applied under make up helps to protect the skin against the elements, while at the same time holding in the skin's natural moisture.

When caring for your face it is easy to forget your neck, especially during the winter when it is often covered up. However you should extend your skin care programme to include this area, or you will find that it ages quickly. To counteract this, use a rich moisturising cream, and keep the area free from make up. Massage your neck with your finger tips in an upward outward motion as you apply the cream.

EXFOLIATION

Another measure in skin care, which is currently increasing in popularity, is exfoliating, or removing the dead surface cells from the skin. This is usually carried out once a week, or twice weekly if the skin looks at all scaly. It involves using a special preparation, which is applied after cleansing, and is then washed or brushed off with a complexion brush. A moisturiser is then applied. Sea salt on a rough wet facecloth can be used for this purpose, but is not recommended for a delicate skin.

HOW TO USE A FACE MASK

A mask applied once or twice a week (depending on skin type – see chart) helps to improve the circulation, and draws out any hidden dirt and toxins. Steaming has a similar effect, but should be avoided by those with sensitive skins, or a tendency to thread veins. You will find some suggestions for suitable face masks in Chapter 11.

Before you apply a mask, cleanse your face, and apply a toner as you would normally. Put the mask on all over your face, but avoid the eye area. Most masks give the best results if they are left on for a period of time (usually up to twenty minutes), and you could treat this as an ideal opportunity to lie down and relax with your feet up.

Remove the mask with warm water, then pat your skin dry and apply your usual toner and moisturiser. Your skin will feel wonderfully smooth and clean. A word of warning though – do not apply a mask a day or two before a special occasion, since it can sometimes draw impurities to the surface of the skin, thus marring your complexion with unwanted spots.

MUSCLE TONE

Facial exercises also have a part to play in improving the complexion, since they serve to stimulate the circulation, tone the muscles, and discourage wrinkle formation. These exercises, which really involve little more than making funny faces, are best practised in seclusion or you'll find yourself getting some very strange looks!

At any time you should try not to tense your facial muscles, since this not only looks unsightly but encourages wrinkles. You'll probably find that whenever you are under stress you tend to tense up certain muscles in your face, and it will take a conscious effort to break this habit.

Here are a few simple face exercises, which can be practised whenever you have a few spare minutes:

1. Open your eyes as wide as you can and count to five.
2. Purse your lips together as if you were going to whistle. Follow this by opening your mouth as wide as you can.
3. Puff out your cheeks as far as you can and count to ten. Expel air rapidly.
4. A good exercise for the neck, which also helps aching shoulders, is to rotate your head all the way round in a circle, stretching your neck as much as possible. Do this three times in each direction.
5. Raise your eyebrows as high as you can, and hold for a count of six.

CARING FOR YOUR BODY

So far we have concentrated on caring for the face, but having given it all this attention, it is important not to neglect the rest of your body.

To delay the ageing process, it is important to keep the skin all over the body well moisturised. The simplest way to do this is to add a moisturising oil or lotion to your bath water, the oil being preferable for drier skins, although it does tend to leave the bath in rather a mess. If you suffer from really dry skin, you should rub in a moisturising body lotion after your bath. Do this while your skin is still warm and slightly damp, so that the moisturiser soaks really well into the skin. This treatment is also to be recommended when you return, sun tanned but dry-skinned, from a holiday.

BATH PREPARATIONS

You can alter the nature of your bath by the ingredients you add to it, and there is no need to spend a lot of money on expensive bath preparations. A good bath oil, for instance, can be made by mixing a cupful of vegetable oil with a teaspoonful of herbal shampoo. Add a few drops of perfume if you like, and beat or blend the ingredients until well mixed. Use about four tablespoonsful of this mixture for each bath.

Bran or oatmeal tied in a muslin cloth and added to the bathwater softens and smoothes the skin. Don't try adding it loose to the bath, though, or you'll have an awful job scraping all the bits off your skin! Use one tablespoonful for a bath. You can also use the cloth as a wash cloth to rub off any rough skin, especially on the heels, knees, elbows, thighs or upper arms. These are areas to pay special attention to, since they can easily become dry and develop the appearance of orange peel. Rub them with a rough cloth or friction mitt whenever you have a bath, and add plenty of moisturiser after drying.

A spoonful of honey added to the bathwater is said to relax and aid sleep, while a bagful of herbs adds a luxurious scent to the water. To soothe aching muscles, soften the skin, and relieve any itchiness, add a cupful of cider vinegar to your bath, and let yourself soak for 15 to 20 minutes. (The smell will soon wear off!). You'll also find other bathtime ideas in Chapter 10.

Remember not to have the water too hot when bathing – 75-80°F is quite hot enough. If you can stand the shock, a cold bath or shower is very invigorating, and helps to stimulate the circulation. After your bath, gently pat and rub yourself dry, before applying your body lotion, talcum powder and deodorant.

CHAPTER FOUR

BEAUTY PROBLEMS

No matter how scrupulously you care for your appearance, there is almost bound to be a time when you are faced with a beauty problem of one sort or another. If it is like most beauty problems, it will probably crop up just when you least want it, like that annoying spot which appears on the very day that you have an important engagement.

Armed with the right information, however, most of the common problems can be overcome with care and perseverance. This chapter sets out some of the more frequent problems, and tells you how to cope with them. You'll also find that the general chapters on caring for your hair/skin/eyes, etc., contain information relevant to such problems as greasy skin or dry hair, so it is worth referring to these too.

ACNE

This is most common during adolescent years, when it is caused at least in part by a hormone imbalance. However, as most of us know to our cost, spots or blackheads can appear at any stage of life, even with those people who have not suffered previously. Spots occur when an excess of oil is secreted by the sebaceous glands, and as it rises to the surface of the skin its exit is blocked by dirt. This causes the sebum to harden and fester, resulting in a spot. Where the tip of this comes into contact with the air it is oxidized and turns black, giving the characteristic blackhead.

First and foremost with acne, the skin must be kept scrupulously clean. The skin should be cleansed two or three times each day using a medicated cleanser, followed by a medicated or pure soap if your skin is also very greasy. Resist the temptation to squeeze spots and blackheads, and touch the infected area as little as possible, ensuring that your hands are clean to prevent the spread of infection. After cleansing apply an astringent, followed by a light liquid moisturiser used very sparingly to counteract any tendency to flakiness. Avoid wearing make up whenever possible.

You should also pay attention to your diet, avoiding fried, starchy or refined foods, chocolate, coffee, carbonated drinks and alcohol. Eat as much fresh fruit and vegetables as you can. A supplement of vitamins B and C is often helpful, as is a daily intake of lecithin. This supplement, which is derived from soya beans, acts as an emulsifier in the body, i.e., it helps to break down and disperse fats. Take two tablespoonsful of lecithin granules, or six capsules, daily. You should also be sure to get plenty of sleep, exercise and fresh air to improve your circulation, and increase the flow of blood to the skin surface.

A face mask two or three times a week helps to heal and draw blemishes to the surface, while at the same time stimulating the circulation and minimizing any open pores. Use a steam facial first, following the instructions in the chart on page 38, since this helps to open the pores. Then apply a mask of natural yogurt, or a mixture of honey and wheat germ, remembering to avoid the delicate eye area. After about twenty minutes, rinse the mask off with warm water, then apply your usual astringent and moisturiser.

AGE SPOTS
This is the unflattering name given to the brown spots which sometimes appear on the backs of the hands. These are attributed to a lack of vitamins E, C and B, so it could be beneficial to take a natural supplement of these vitamins.

Bleaching sometimes helps the spots to disappear – try equal parts of cider vinegar, distilled water and milk, or equal parts of lemon juice and rosewater. Pat on to the affected area, and leave on for between fifteen minutes and several hours. Wash off with tepid water, pat dry, and apply an astringent followed by a rich moisturising cream.

DANDRUFF

This is usually one of two different types: dry or oily. The presence of either form suggests an imbalance in the body, often due to faulty diet. Dry dandruff is usually concentrated around the ears and the hair line, and can be very itchy. Many factors are thought to contribute to dandruff, such as emotional tension, poor health, harsh shampoos, exposure to cold, and general tiredness.

It is important to keep the hair and scalp clean to minimize the accumulation of dead cells. Brush the hair daily to improve the circulation and remove any flakiness. Another daily habit to acquire is to massage the scalp thoroughly, using your fingertips and working systematically all over the head (see instructions on page 50). Extra benefit can be achieved if you apply a herbal tonic before your daily massage. Steep a handful of herbs such as nettle or rosemary in a pint of boiling water, and leave to stand for up to three hours. Strain, and comb through your hair before massaging. This same tonic can be used as a final rinse after shampooing.

Another measure which helps to counteract dandruff is to dilute cider vinegar with an equal quantity of water, and dab this on to the hair with cotton wool in between shampooing. Cider vinegar added to the final rinsing water after shampooing also helps to disperse dandruff.

As far as diet is concerned, it is important to eat plenty of fresh raw fruit and vegetables, and to drink as much water as you can. At the same time, avoid fatty foods, sugar and refined carbohydrates.

THINNING OR FALLING HAIR

Every day we shed between 40 and 100 hairs, but in the normal way these are replaced by new growth. However, certain illnesses or stages in life can cause more hair than usual to be lost, for instance after having a baby, or in middle age.

To minimize this hair loss, check that you are eating the right foods for healthy hair (see page 54). Particularly important are the B vitamins, which are best supplied by brewer's yeast, wholemeal bread, liver, wheat germ, and wholegrains. Take a daily brewer's yeast supplement, either in the form of powder, or tablets (up to six daily).

Although you may be reluctant to touch your head for fear of aggravating the hair loss, daily massage is essential to stimulate the scalp circulation and promote new growth. Try gently pulling the hair too, but only when it is dry since any pressure on wet hair will stretch and break it. The nettle tonic recommended for dandruff can be used in conjunction with massage as a means of stimulating hair growth. If you have long hair, change the position of your parting regularly to prevent strain on the roots, which could stop the follicles from producing new hair. For the same reason, don't keep your hair tied back in a pony tail for long periods.

Always use warm as opposed to hot water for washing the hair, avoiding the use of harsh detergent shampoos. Try a soap-based one, or a mild baby shampoo instead. It is best to let your hair dry naturally, and not to use rollers of any kind. If you feel you must set your hair, tie several layers of tissues around the rollers, or use foam ones which are gentler on the hair.

Tension is also said to be a factor in hair loss, and it is the increased stresses of life today which are blamed for the fact that many women are now showing a tendency to baldness. So, learn how to relax.

FACIAL HAIR

This is a problem encountered by many women, and is particularly common during the menopause. The hair is usually to be found above the upper lip, or on the sides of the face.

There are several methods of removing facial hair, and the one you choose depends very much on the severity of the problem. Plucking should be considered only if there are one or two stray hairs. Bleaching is suitable only for very fine, downy hair. Use a very diluted solution of peroxide, but test it first on the back of your hand in case it causes an allergic reaction. Any form of bleach tends to dry the skin, so use plenty of nourishing cream afterwards.

Some depilatory creams are produced specifically for facial hair, but as with the bleach, do an allergy test before embarking. The only permanent method of removing hair is electrolysis, a method in which the hair root is cauterized by giving it a tiny electric shock. The success of this treatment depends on the skill of the operator, so always ensure that a reputable salon is chosen. Unskilled electrolysis could result in nasty scarring.

GREY HAIR

This is largely determined by heredity – and there is nothing you can do about that! However, premature greyness can be delayed by increasing scalp circulation, and by ensuring an abundance of certain nutrients in the diet. Tests have shown that foods rich in iodine, iron, copper, vitamins B and F can help restore colour to greying hair, but any improvements is likely to be visible only after a good few months. Pantothenic acid, PABA (*P*-aminobenzoic acid) and folic acid are the three B vitamins said to restore colour. If you want to try a treatment, said by one American doctor to have a 70 per cent success rate, take a daily supplement of 100mg PABA, 30mg calcium pantothenate, and 2 grammes of choline. Since these are all present in brewer's yeast, this may be the simplest way to supplement.

EYE WRINKLES

As you will read in the chapter on eyes, the skin in this area is so delicate that it is one of the first to wrinkle, especially if maltreated. You should follow the general advice given in that chapter, but in addition try using an eye cream containing vitamin E (such as that on page 82). This vitamin is said to delay and minimize wrinkles if used consistently over a period of time, but remember to apply the cream correctly (see page 57), or you will simply aggravate the problem.

THREAD VEINS

These are particularly common in those with a dry or sensitive skin. Once acquired they are difficult to eradicate, but you can help prevent them from growing worse by increasing your daily vitamin C intake (i.e., plenty of fresh raw fruit and vegetables, especially citrus fruits, blackcurrants, and green peppers). This is because these broken veins are believed to be caused by lack of vitamin C in the diet.

Try to avoid tea, coffee and alcohol, each of which aggravates the condition. Drink herb teas instead. You can make these yourself in the same way that you would make ordinary tea, using 1 teaspoonful dried or 3 teaspoonsful fresh herb per person, plus one for the pot. Pour on boiling water and leave to stand for 5 minutes before drinking. Coltsfoot is particularly suitable.

It is important to avoid extremes of temperature. Use only warm water when washing, and protect the skin with a moisturiser before venturing out in cold or hot weather. Steam facials should also be avoided.

In severe cases thread veins can be treated by electrolysis, which is used to dry up the tiny veins. There is nothing this treatment can do to prevent fresh outbreaks elsewhere though. A marigold lotion, made from the flowers infused in boiling water (follow the instructions for nettle tonic on page 33), can help if patted on to the affected area each day after cleansing. It is also worth rubbing the face with the inside peel of citrus fruit.

YOUR SKIN CARE CHART

Skin Type	How to Recognize	Cleanse	Tone
Normal	Smooth, soft and fine textured. The occasional spot but no real problems. In fact it's a very rare skin type.	Light cleansing cream, or a rinse-off cleanser with water. Eye make up remover for delicate eye area.	Light skin tonic.
Greasy	Face quickly becomes shiny. Tissue held to skin looks greasy. Prone to open pores and blemishes, especially around nose.	2-3 times daily use a medicated cleaner or a rinse-off cleaner.	Apply astringent, paying particular attention to greasiest areas like sides of nose, chin and forehead.
Dry	Flaky and dull, especially round eyes and on cheeks. Feels taut after using soap, and becomes red and sore in cold weather.	Massage in rich cleansing cream, and wipe off with cotton wool. Avoid using tap water – if necessary use creamy face wash and mineral water once a day.	Very gentle toner, avoiding upper cheeks. Dilute toner if skin is very dry.
Combi-nation	A greasy panel down centre of face, with dryish areas on cheeks and around eyes.	Use a light cream, especially on greasy areas. Follow this with a rinse-off cleanser or soap on greasy areas only.	Light toning lotion, followed by astringent on greasy areas.

Moisturise	Special Treatment	Diet
Light liquid moisturiser night and morning. A light eye cream at night. Light throat cream.	Weekly mask or light steam facial. Use the latter only if no thread veins. Add a handful of rosemary or chamomile to 1 pt. (550ml) boiling water. Put face about 12 inches above bowl, cover head, and remain for 5 minutes. Finish with toner and moisturiser.	Plenty of fresh raw fruit and vegetables, protein and wholegrains.
A light liquid moisturiser especially on cheeks. Eye and neck creams.	Twice a week use a mask or steam facial with rosemary or sage. Finish with an astringent.	Avoid fatty or fried food, chocolate, tea, coffee, and alcohol. Eat plenty of green vegetables.
Light moisturiser during the day, with a rich nourishing cream at night. Use this on neck as well. Apply eye cream each night too.	Moisturising facial once weekly, e.g. honey, avocado or egg yolk. Leave on for up to 20 minutes, then wipe off, tone and moisturise.	Include unsaturated fats in the form of vegetable oils and nuts. Get plenty of vitamins A, B complex, C and E.
Liquid moisturiser all over face, followed by rich nourishing cream on dry areas.	Once a week face mask, using one of the suggestions for dry skin on cheeks, and egg white and lemon juice on greasy centre panel.	As for normal skin, but restrict greasy foods.

CHAPTER FIVE

A SENSIBLE APPROACH TO SLIMMING

Obesity and beauty definitely don't go together. It's hard to look beautiful when you're bulging in all the wrong places, although it's not just your face and figure which are affected when you are carrying excess weight. Your self-confidence suffers a severe blow too – and pride in your appearance plays an important part in being beautiful.

If you are overweight you are also placing an extra strain on your heart, and as a result you run an increased risk of falling prey to such severe ailments as corony heart disease, high blood pressure or diabetes.

Getting your figure in trim is therefore one of the first steps to take, for the sake of both your looks and your health. You need not think that you have to be wafer thin to be beautiful. In recent years we have become diet crazy (hardly surprising, perhaps, when it is estimated that one in five adults in Britain are overweight), and there must be almost as many diets as there are overweight people.

Some of these diets are so severe and extreme that they are likely to be more detrimental to your health than being overweight. Crash diets which severely restrict food intake or exclude all but one or two food items are not to be recommended, however serious your obesity problem. Not only is your health likely to suffer, but if you do succeed in adhering to such a diet and losing weight, you are likely to put many of those lost pounds back on again once you resume your normal eating habits.

There is a risk with most slimming diets that in cutting down on the amount of food you eat, you are also drastically reducing your intake of vital nutrients. When this happens you are likely to suffer from the tiredness and irritability so familiar to slimmers. The only sensible way to lose weight (and to maintain that weight loss) is to follow a carefully balanced diet which makes up in quality for what you lose in quantity.

WHOLEFOODS

This is where wholefoods come into their own. Because they retain a higher proportion of nutrients than refined foods, you are getting more goodness from the food you eat. Wholefoods not only supply more vitamins and minerals than refined foods; their natural roughage also aids the digestion, and makes the foods more satisfying so that you need eat less. Those following a high fibre diet have also been shown to absorb approximately ten per cent fewer calories from their food than those on a low fibre diet.

Wholefoods are not specifically slimming foods, but their extra nutritional value means that you stay happy and healthy while you slim. A wholefood diet also includes plenty of fresh fruit and vegetables, which add extra variety and goodness but very few calories. Readjusting your eating habits along wholefood lines should not be regarded as a temporary measure though. Eating the wholefood way will help you to stay slim and healthy even when you have reached your ideal weight.

Using the calorie chart and food list included in this chapter, you can work out a wholefood diet to suit yourself, bearing in mind that to achieve an appreciable weight loss, women should follow a 1000 calorie diet, and men a 1500 calorie diet. For those who prefer to follow a more rigid diet plan, a seven day wholefood diet is also included. This was devised by *Slimming Naturally*, a magazine catering for those who want to lose weight and stay healthy.

Whatever diet you choose, the following points are worth bearing in mind while you are slimming:

Cut down the amount of fat you eat to about 1 oz.

(25g) a day. Do not totally exclude fat from your diet or your skin and hair will pay the penalty. Ideally, the fat you use should be in the form of unsaturated vegetable oil or margarine, but don't on any account use these for frying or your calorie count will go shooting up.

Keep your fluid intake to a minimum, since drinking excess fluid can aggravate problems of overweight by causing fluid retention. Restrict tea and coffee to two cups a day or, better still, cut them out completely. Cut right back as well on your alcohol intake while slimming. Herb teas have no calories at all (provided you add no sweetening), and some are useful to slimmers since they are both diaphoretic (promoting sweating) and diuretic. Choose peppermint, mace, rosehip or dandelion. Lemon juice also acts as a diuretic, and, as can be seen from the seven day diet, can be taken for this purpose first thing in the morning with hot water.

Make up quantities of skim milk powder to use in place of whole milk for drinks and cooking. It's much lower in calories.

If you must eat between meals, choose raw fruit or vegetables from the free list.

Cook all food carefully to retain maximum nutrient content, without increasing the calories. This means eating vegetables raw, or lightly boiled or steamed.Grill meat wherever possible, and pour away the cooking juices when roasting since these are high in fat.

Watch out for nutritious but high calorie foods such as nuts, hard cheeses, commercial fruit yogurt, avocado pears, and alcohol.

Include lots of salads in your diet (they are low in calories and a good source of vitamins and minerals), but avoid high calorie dressings. Instead, try one of the following: half a carton natural yogurt with the juice of half a lemon, and a dash of honey and mustard; large spoonful of milk powder, mixed with a spoonful each of cider vinegar and lemon juice (add a spoonful of curry powder for spicy flavour); half a cupful of tomato juice with the juice of half a lemon and a teaspoon of chopped onion, chives or garlic.

Unfortunately, no easy, painless way of losing weight has yet been discovered. Whatever diet or slimming aids you use, it's still a question of will power – without it, you're fighting a losing battle! However, there are some foods which can be included in a wholefood diet to speed your weight loss, and to keep you happy and healthy while you're slimming.

THE WONDER COMBINATION –
Lecithin/Cider Vinegar/Kelp/Vitamin B6

Top of this list must come four health food ingredients which, when taken in combination, have been found by slimmers to speed up weight loss. These foods, of course, will not lead to loss of weight on their own, but must be taken in conjunction with a low calorie diet.

The Lecithin/Cider Vinegar/Kelp/Vitamin B6 low calorie diet was first discovered by an American journalist called Mary Ann Crenshaw. She labelled the four special ingredients 'fat fighters' and she introduced the diet to readers of her book *The Natural Way to Super Beauty*, published in America in 1974. As a result, dieters on both sides of the Atlantic were soon following her example. Indeed, the diet has become so popular that manufacturers are now producing slimming capsules which combine all these four elements in the correct proportions in an easy-to-take form. Such capsules are readily available from health food shops, and they are proving to be a continuing best seller.

It was whilst researching nutritional theory and experimenting with strict 1000 calorie diets that Mary Ann Crenshaw discovered that, for her, these four 'fat fighters' worked wonders. She says in her book that after using them in her low-calorie regimen for two weeks she lost a full 12 lb in weight, and she also found that her new diet worked just as well on her friends.

Consistent with what is said above, she emphasizes in her book that her Lecithin/Cider Vinegar/Kelp/Vitamin B6 formula is not a miracle slim system by itself. Your diet is the important thing if you wish to lose weight and stay slim, but as she says: '… my four little friends sure did make things easier. And quicker, which is the best part of all.' It is good to know, too, that these four ingredients are not drugs but foods.

Mary Ann Crenshaw worked out her diet on the basis of the following theories:

Lecithin is present in every cell in the human body, and it also occurs naturally in egg yolks, some vegetable oils and soya beans. Lecithin acts as an emulsifier, which means that it breaks up fat and so helps to prevent it accumulating in the body. It also acts as a natural diuretic, and is one of the best sources of two hard to get B vitamins, choline and inositol, both of which are important to hair health. As a food supplement, lecithin is usually derived from soya beans and is available in either granular or capsule form. Mary Ann Crenshaw took one to two tablespoonsful of lecithin granules daily on her diet, this amount being equivalent to three British teaspoonsful.

Cider Vinegar is a rich source of many of the minerals, and appears to have a regulating effect on the body metabolism. It has been credited with the ability to relieve a wide variety of ailments, especially arthritis and rheumatism, and throat and bronchial complaints. Mary Ann Crenshaw included it in her diet as a rich source of the mineral potassium, which encourages the body to excrete excess fluid. For the purpose of slimming, take a teaspoonful of cider vinegar in a glass of water with every meal.

Kelp is the name given to a dried seaweed, which is used as a food supplement because it is one of the richest known sources of minerals, particularly iodine. This is the mineral needed by the thyroid gland, which controls the body metabolism and therefore determines how quickly food is burned up. Women are more likely to be deficient in iodine than men, and a shortage is particularly common during adolescence and youth. Mary Ann Crenshaw, who put on weight easily and knew that she had a slow metabolism, took 200 milligrammes of kelp each day.

Vitamin B6, also known as pyrodoxine, is the member of the B complex which is essential to the nervous system, and the first signs of a deficiency are irritability and depression. Women taking the Pill are especially likely to be short of this vitamin. B6 also appears to balance the levels of potassium and sodium in the body, which means that it helps counteract fluid retention. Mary Ann Crenshaw took 50 milligrammes a day.

Other wholefoods which will assist the slimmer in his or her battle against overweight include the following:

BRAN
A valuable source of roughage, and as such will ward off the constipation which is so often experienced by slimmers. The normal amount to take is up to two tablespoonsful daily, the exact amount required varying from one person to another. A teaspoonful of bran taken in liquid before meals also helps to take the edge off the appetite, so that you are inclined to eat less. Bran, which comes in a finely flaked form, can be added to cereals or desserts, drinks, savoury dishes or used in baking.

WHEAT GERM
Like bran, this is removed during the manufacture of white flour and is prized as a rich source of vitamins E, B, and A, as well as being 28 per cent protein. Also present are quantities of unsaturated fats and

minerals. Wheat germ can be sprinkled on cereals, mixed into casseroles, soups or drinks, or included in baking. It also makes a good substitute for breadcrumbs, or can be eaten alone with milk or yogurt.

BREWER'S YEAST
Not only a rich source of protein, but also contains the B complex vitamins, and fourteen minerals. It's an excellent pick-me-up, and comes in the form of tablets or powder. The strong taste of the latter is best disguised by adding it to soups, drinks, casseroles or cereals.

SKIM MILK POWDER
As already mentioned, this is much lower in calories than whole milk. It is also free from fat, and is a good source of protein, calcium, and many of the B vitamins. As well as being used as a substitute for whole milk, a spoonful of the powder can be added to other foods to boost their nutrient content.

THE A TO Z OF WHOLEFOOD CALORIES
All calorie amounts are approximate, and are given per ounce of food.

Beans (cooked)			*Breakfast cereals*	
Butter	26		Flaked cereals	100-110
Haricot	25		Granola cereals	130-140
Lentils	27		Grapenuts	100
			Muesli	100-110
Biscuits			Oats, uncooked	112
Oatcakes	100		Porridge, cooked	13
Savoury biscuits	120-140		Puffed cereals	100
Sweet biscuits	120-140		Wheat biscuits	100-106
Bran			*Cakes*	100-140
Bran cereals	90-100			
Miller's bran	92		*Carob flour*	51
Bread			*Cheese*	
Granary, white or brown	70-73		Cottage	30-33
Wholemeal	64		Cream	232

Curd	39
Edam	90
Other hard cheeses	100-120

Cream	
Double	131
Single	62

Crispbreads	per slice
Biscottes	30-35
Starch reduced slices	21-24
Primula Rye	17
Kelloggs Scanda Brod brown	32
Scanda Crisp	19
Ryvita	26
Rye King	28
brown	35

Dried Fruit	
Apple rings	71
Apricots	52
Currants	69
Dates	70
Figs	61
Prunes	46
Seeded raisins	80
Sultanas	71

Eggs	46

Fats and Oils	
Butter and margarine	226
Oils	262

Fish	
Oily (tuna, herring, mackerel, sardine)	65-85
Salmon, tinned	36
Shellfish	30
White fish	18-30

Flour and Grains	
Uncooked wholegrains, and the flours into	
which they are ground range from	95-105

Fruit, fresh	
Apples, grapes, cherries	14
Avocado pear	25
Banana	22
Grapefruit, melon, soft fruit	6
Lemons, gooseberries	4
Oranges, peaches	10
Pear, pineapple, plum	12
Tangerines, apricots	8

Fruit bars (per bar)	90-160

Ice Cream	50

Juices, unsweetened	
Apple	10
Carrot, grapefruit, orange, lemon	12
Grape	19
Pineapple	16
Tomato, vegetable	6

Meat, fresh (lean only)	
Beef	49
Chicken, veal	31
Duck, rabbit	42
Kidney (raw, lamb's)	28
Lamb, turkey	40
Liver	38
Minced beef	80
Pork	54

Milk	
Buttermilk	11
Dried powder (made up)	10
Evaporated	49
Soya liquid	10
Whole, liquid	18

Nuts, shelled	
Almonds	164
Brazil	180
Cashew, coconut	178

Chestnut	49	Molasses	73
Hazel	108	All sugars	112
Peanuts	166		
Walnuts	151	*Vegetables, fresh*	
Chopped, mixed	148	Aubergine (raw),	
Mixed nuts and		green beans,	
raisins	109	broccoli, spinach	
Peanut butter	180	(raw), courgette	
		(raw), watercress, radish	4
Nutmeats		Broad beans, beetroot	13
Granose Nutbrawn	37	Chicory, cucumber,	
Meatless Steaks	36	lettuce	3
Nutmeat	57	Carrots, onions, swedes,	
Nuttolene	87	turnips	6
Prewett's Brazilia Mix	117	Cauliflower, cabbage,	
Rissol-nut	129	spring greens, bean	
Sausalatas	36	sprouts, asparagus	8
		Leeks	9
Pasta, cooked	32	Mushrooms (raw),	2
		Parsnips	14
Salad dressings		Peas	20
Mayonnaise	202	Peppers,	10
Salad cream	108	Brussels sprouts	24
		Potatoes	
Seeds, shelled		Sweetcorn	28
Linseed, sunflower	170	Tomatoes fresh	4
Pumpkin	155	canned	43
Sesame	161		
		Wheat germ	100
Sugar and sweeteners			
Black treacle	75	*Yogurt*	
Honey	82-90	Low fat, unflavoured	12-16
Jam	80	Fruit flavoured	22

THE SEVEN DAY WHOLEFOOD DIET

Free list	Permitted in small amounts		Occasional treat	
Fresh fruit:	*Fresh raw*		*Seeds:*	
Grapefruit	*vegetables:*		Linseed	170
Soft fruit,	Peas	18	Pumpkin	155
e.g., Blackberries	Potatoes	24	Sesame	161
Melon 6			Sunflower	170
Orange	*Fresh fruit:*			
Peaches 10	Apples		*Nuts:*	
Pears	Grapes		Peanuts	166

Free list		Permitted in small amounts		Occasional treat	
Pineapple		Cherries	14	Cashew	178
Plums	12			Almonds	164
Rhubarb	2	*Meat:*			
Tangerines	8	Grilled gammon	83	Sweet or savoury wholewheat biscuits or cakes	100-140
Fresh raw vegetables:		Beef (grilled lean steak)	86		
Lettuce		Chicken (roast)	54		
Mushrooms		Liver (stewed)	43	*Meat:*	
Celery		Turkey (roast)	56	Duck (roast)	55
Broccoli		Veal cutlet	56	Lamb (roast)	83
Green beans				Pork (roast)	90
Spinach	2	*Meatless meats:*		Rissol-nut	129
Swedes		Meatless steak (TVP)	36		
Tomatoes				*Fats and oils:*	
Turnips	4	Nutmeat	57	Butter	211
Carrots				Margarine	211
Onions	6	*Fish:*		Oils	255
Asparagus		White fish, e.g., cod	20	Soyanutta	266
Cabbage					
Cauliflower		Salmon (tinned)	36	*Sugar and sweeteners:*	
Greens	8	Shellfish	30 (av)	all sugar including	
Broad beans				Fructose	12
Beetroot		Oily fish, e.g., tuna, mackerel, herring, sardine	65-70	Molasses	73
Parsnips	13				
				Others:	
Fruit juices:				Mayonnaise	202
Apple	10			Jams (natural)	80
Grape	19	*Cheese:*		Chutney	20-40
Tomato		Cottage, (low-fat plain)	30-33	Single cream	51
Vegetable (e.g., V8)	6			Fruit bars	90-160
Carrot	12	Hard, e.g., cheddar	100-110	Pasta	32
Grapefruit	16			Granola cereals	130
Orange	14				
Pineapple	16	*Beans, cooked:*		Dry white wine	21
		Butter	26	Draught bitter	9
Crispbreads:		Haricot	25		
Primula Rye extra thin	17	Lentils	27		
Scanda Crisp	19				
		Dried fruit:			
Bran	92	Apple rings	71		
		Apricots	54		

Free list	Permitted in small amounts		Occasional treat
Yeast extract 2	Currants	72	
	Dates	74	
Herbs (for	Figs	54	
seasoning	Prunes	38	
and teas) 0	Seedless		
	raisins	94	
Fresh skimmed	Sultanas	74	
milk, or recon-			
stituted	*Cereals:*		
dried (20 fl.	Muesli base	110	
oz. in one	Porridge		
pint) 10	(made with		
yogurt 15	water and salt)	13	
	Wholegrain		
	boiled rice	95-105	
	Wholewheat		
	bread	64	
	Others:		
	Eggs	45	
	Outline low-		
	fat spread	105	
	Honey	82-90	
	Fresh whole		
	milk	19	

Figures given are calories per ounce (25g).

MENU SUGGESTIONS

Day One   *Calorie count*

On rising:
Cupful hot water and fresh lemon juice   0

Breakfast:
4 oz. (100g) porridge (made with water)   52
2 oz. (50g) grilled gammon and 1 tomato   188
                                                   ———
                                                   240

Lunch:
3 oz. (75g) mixed salad from any vegetables
   on free list   20
2 oz. (50g) cottage cheese   60

1 large slice wholemeal bread spread thinly with margarine	150	
1 fresh fruit, e.g., orange	40	
1 cup hot yeast extract	0	
		270

Supper:

4 oz. (100g) any white fish wrapped in foil, with mushrooms, a little lemon juice, salt, herbs and $\frac{1}{2}$ oz. ($12\frac{1}{2}$g) margarine	185	
3 oz. (75g) vegetables from free list	18	
1 fresh fruit, e.g., apple sliced with 1 oz. (25g) natural yogurt	55	
4 oz. (100g) baked jacket potato	96	

Total calories for day: 354

864

Day Two

On rising:

Cupful hot water and fresh lemon juice	0

Breakfast:

Poached egg	90	
Slice wholemeal toast and margarine	75	
Grilled tomato	4	169

Lunch:

6 oz. (175g) salad (from free list)	40	
1 oz. (25g) low fat natural yogurt as dressing	20	
3 oz. (75g) sardines (drained of oil)	195	
1 peach	20	275

Supper:

Vegetable soup (any on free list made with yeast extract stock and seasoned with herbs)	70	
4 oz. (100g) cauliflower with cheese sauce made from 1oz. cheddar and $\frac{1}{4}$ pt. (150ml) low fat skimmed milk, served with grilled tomato, and baked potato plus knob of butter	250	
5 oz. (150g) cubed melon	30	350

Total calories for day: 794

Day Three
On rising:

Cupful hot water and fresh lemon juice	0

Breakfast:

2 oz. (50g) stewed prunes or apricots	45	
4 oz. (100g) natural low fat yogurt	60	
1 tablespoonful bran	18	
1 slice wholemeal toast spread thinly with margarine	75	
		198

Lunch:

Salad Nicoise made with 1 hard boiled egg, 1 tomato, 2-3 anchovy fillets, 3-4 black olives, 2 oz. (50g) cooked green beans, lemon juice and herb dressing	106	
1 apple	38	
1 oz. (25g) cheddar cheese	100	
		244

Supper:

Ratatouille made with vegetables from free list, and baked with 1 oz. (25g) oil	142	
2 oz. (50g) roast chicken	108	
1 large eating pear sliced and served with spicy lemon sauce made as follows: combine juice of one lemon with pinch ginger and pinch cinnamon. Heat for two minutes and leave to cool. Pour over pear and chill for ten minutes.	45	
		295
Total calories for day:		754

Day Four
On rising:

Cupful hot water and fresh lemon juice	0

Breakfast:

Half grapefruit	24	
1 boiled egg with wholemeal bread	210	
		234

Lunch:

1 large baked potato filled with cottage cheese and chives and knob of butter	200	
1 oz. (25g) grapes	14	
		214

Supper:

2 oz. (50g) raw mushrooms served with 3 oz. (75g) natural yogurt and little chopped raw onion	50
2 oz. (50g) liver stewed with tomatoes, onions, herbs, and served with 4 oz. (100g) broccoli	110
1 apple baked with ½ oz. (12½g) raisins	89
	249
Total calories for day:	697

Day Five:

On rising:

Cupful hot water and fresh lemon juice	0

Breakfast:

1 large egg scrambled with ½ oz. (12½g) butter	202
1 slice wholemeal bread and margarine	75
	277

Lunch:

4 crispbread spread with banana and date	152
2 oz. (50g) plain yogurt with 3 oz. (75g) raspberries	52
	204

Supper:

2 oz. (50g) boiled wholegrain rice mixed with 1 small pepper fried in ½ teaspoonful oil and seasoned with herbs and soy sauce, topped with 1 oz. (25g) grated cheese:	370
3 oz. (75g) blackberries	18
	388
Total calories for day:	869

Day Six

On rising:

Cup hot water and fresh lemon juice	0

Breakfast:

4 oz. (100g) porridge made with water	52
1 poached egg, 1 tomato and 1 oz. (25g) grilled mushrooms	104
	156

Lunch:

Apple cheese and celery salad, made with 4 oz. (100g) cottage cheese, 2 sticks celery and 2 oz. (50g) apple	156
4 crispbread	35
	191

Supper:

Kebabs: put alternately on skewers pepper, onion, tomato, mushrooms	42
Served with 2 oz. (50g) wholegrain rice	200
4 dessert plums with 1 oz. (25g) single cream	91
	333
Total calories for day:	**680**

Day Seven

On rising:

Cupful hot water and fresh lemon juice	0

Breakfast:

As Day 3, without toast	123
	123

Lunch:

1 oz. (25g) vegetable or liver pâté	97
2 slices wholemeal bread	123
3 oz. (75g) salad from free list	20
	240

Supper:

Three sticks celery, braised in vegetable stock for 30 minutes	10
1 large baked potato with 1 oz. (25g) grated cheese and ½ oz. (12½g) butter	280
4 oz. (100g) mixed fruit salad from free list, with lemon juice and a little honey	60
	350
Total calories for day:	**713**

N.B. menus allow for 200 calories to be used on drinks.

CHAPTER SIX

HAIR CARE

If you are one of those people whose idea of hair care begins and ends with a quick shampoo once or twice a week, you have a lot to learn. Very few people give their hair the care and attention it needs – which is no doubt why it is so common to see hair that shows obvious signs of neglect. Certainly the sleek, shining locks one sees in glossy magazines seem to be a long way removed from everyday life.

Before you can begin to care for your hair, it helps to have at least a basic knowledge of its structure. The hair is composed of a protein-based substance called keratin – the same substance which forms finger and toe nails. Each hair consists of three layers, the central core or medulla being made up of spongy tissues which may contain some colour pigment. This is surrounded by the middle layer, the cortex, which consists of long thin cells that give the hair its elasticity and colour. The outer hair layer, known as the cuticle, consists of hundreds of tiny, overlapping scales.

Hair grows from the hair follicle, which is an enclosed sac situated below the surface of the scalp. The follicles, which contain the hair roots, are fed by blood carrying nutrients, hence the importance of good circulation to healthy hair. It is the supply of nutrients which determines the health of the hair as it emerges from the scalp and continues to grow. Hair grows at the rate of about half an inch a month, although this speeds up somewhat during summer, and slows down with age. Once hair leaves the follicle it is in fact technically 'dead', but it grows because of continued tissue formation within the follicle.

Halfway along the hair follicle are located the sebaceous glands which secrete the oil that gives healthy hair its natural sheen. It is a disturbance in the production of sebum by these glands which results in hair that is over dry or greasy.

Both your natural hair colour, and whether it is straight or curly, are determined by heriditary factors. In those who have curly hair, it is the actual shape of the hair follicle which forces the emerging hair to develop waves.

FOODS FOR HEALTHY HAIR
As mentioned above, the necessary nutrients must be available if you are to have healthy hair. The advice contained in Chapter 2 applies equally to hair and skin, but there are also certain nutrients of particular importance to hair health. The B complex vitamins, for instance, influence hair growth, oil production and colour, so an ample supply of these is essential. Vitamins A and C also have a part to play in the production of healthy hair. Since the hair is formed from keratin, which is itself a protein-like substance, the diet also needs to include adequate quantities of protein in the form of meat, fish, dairy produce, pulses or nuts. Of the minerals, copper, iron and iodine are essential to healthy hair. Copper is widely available in food, while liver, kidneys, wholegrains and molasses are good sources of iron. The only foods that contain appreciable quantities of iodine are seafoods.

Your hair, like your skin, is affected not only by diet and health, but also by tension. In a person who is tense the muscles at the base of the neck are constricted, and this impedes the flow of blood to the scalp, resulting in weak hair growth.

WHAT HAIR CARE REALLY MEANS
Another characteristic which hair shares with skin is that it will fall into one of three categories, namely

dry, greasy or normal. The care you give your hair will be influenced by its type, but as with skin care there are certain basic guidelines which apply to all types.

A mistake people often make is to wash their hair too frequently, when in fact this is likely to do more harm than good. Shampoos may make hair clean, but at the same time they remove its natural oils and protective acid coating.

A shampoo once a week is enough for most hair, and even very greasy hair should not be washed any more frequently than is absolutely necessary. The temptation to wash greasy hair every couple of days should be resisted, since the more you wash it, the more you stimulate the already over-active sebaceous glands. In other words, all you will do is end up with even greasier hair. If you get desperate, try using bran or oatmeal as a dry shampoo. Just rub well into the hair, and then brush out thoroughly. Eau de cologne or lavender water sprinkled on to a piece of cheesecloth or nylon stocking and stretched over a hairbrush also helps to remove dirt and grease between shampoos.

While on the subject of brushes, that old idea of a hundred brush strokes a day is just as valid now as ever. Regular brushing not only stimulates the scalp circulation, but also serves to distribute the natural oils from the scalp all along the hair to its tip. Brushing helps, too, to remove any flakiness which may accumulate. Make sure, though, that you use a natural bristle brush and not a nylon one which tends to stretch and split the hair. Keep your brush clean by washing it each week. When giving your hair its daily brush, lean the head forwards and brush from the nape of the neck towards the forehead. If your hair is at all tangled, a wide toothed comb is gentler than a brush.

Make just before or after brushing the time when you treat yourself to a scalp massage. Like brushing, this stimulates the circulation, dislodges dirt and dandruff, and encourages hair growth. To give yourself a massage, spread your fingers fanwise and slip them through the hair. With your thumbs pressed behind your ears, press down on your scalp with your fingertips. Now rotate your fingers so that they move the scalp over the bony structure of the head – you'll feel your skin move and the scalp tingle. Move up an inch at a time until you have covered the whole head. This sounds rather complicated, but in fact it is a very simple procedure, and takes only a few minutes to perform. Massage your scalp daily if you find the time, or at the very least once a week (this is especially important for those suffering from dandruff or falling hair).

THE RIGHT WAY TO WASH YOUR HAIR
When washing your hair, always use warm not hot water. Once your hair is wet, apply just a small quantity of shampoo and work gently into the hair using a circular motion. It is this massaging of the scalp which encourages good circulation, as well as ensuring that the hair is really clean. After shampooing give your hair a really good rinse to remove all traces of soap. Only if your hair is really dirty does it need a second application of shampoo. If you can bear it, the final rinse should be with cool water since this helps to close the pores.

Whatever your hair type, the shampoo you choose is of the utmost importance. The best ones to use are natural or herbal since these contain less harsh detergents, and have the added bonus of hair helpers like nettle, rosemary or chamomile. Hair has a natural acid coating which will become unbalanced if the shampoo you use is too harsh or alkaline. The acid/alkaline balance is measured on a scale indicated by a pH number, a pH balanced shampoo being between 5 and 8 on the scale. The acidity of a shampoo is particularly important for hair that is coloured or permed, since both these practices leave an acid residue.

CONDITIONING

The time to apply a hair conditioner is after your hair is thoroughly cleansed. These products are especially helpful for long hair, where the overlapping scales which cover the outer layer of hair often get roughed up as it grows. A conditioner helps to smooth these scales down, and to give shining hair which is easier to comb and manage. hair that is coloured, permed, or exposed to sun also benefits from a conditioner. In the normal way, dry hair should be conditioned once a week, normal hair once a fortnight, and greasy hair not more than once a month.

After conditioning, rinse your hair again, adding cider vinegar or lemon juice to the rinse water to remove all vestiges of soap, and to restore the hair's natural acid coating. Lemon juice is usually used on blonde hair since it acts as a mild bleach.

When your hair is wet, always use a comb, since brushing will stretch and tear it. Start with the ends of the hair, and work up towards the scalp. The kindest way to dry your hair is naturally, but if you want to use a hair dryer always have it on the coolest setting since heat dries out the hair. Heated hair rollers or curling tongs also tend to damage the hair, so keep these for use before special occasions only.

If you want to use rollers, choose sponge ones, or wrap ordinary rollers in several layers of toilet paper or tissues to prevent them tearing the hair. Lemon juice combed through the hair after rinsing acts as a natural setting lotion, or you can add gelatine to the final rinse water.

It goes without saying that your hair will never look good unless it is really well cut. Good hairdressers are hard to find, so if you know one stick with him. Unless you have very definite ideas about the style you want, you are best to put yourself in his hands – a good hairdresser will give you a style that not only takes account of your face shape, but also your height, weight, manner of dress, etc.

SOME NATURAL HAIR CARE PRODUCTS

If you suffer from dry hair, a conditioner used after shampooing will, as already mentioned, put some life and lustre back into your hair. An occasional oil treatment also helps improve dry hair. To use this, apply a warmed vegetable oil to your hair, massage it well in, and wrap your head in a towel which has been wrung out in hot water. Leave this on for at least quarter of an hour before shampooing. Cider vinegar or lemon juice in the final rinse water will help to remove any last traces of oil.

An egg yolk shampoo is a gentle cleanser which is especially suited to dry hair. Simply mix one or two egg yolks (depending on the length of your hair) with a little warm water. Make sure the water is not too hot when you add it, or you'll end up with scrambled egg! Apply this mixture to your hair, wrap your head in a towel, and leave for several minutes before rinsing thoroughly. There is no need to apply any other shampoo.

Eggs can also be used as the basis of a protein treatment, which helps restore condition to any hair type. Beat together two eggs, one tablespoonful vegetable oil, one tablespoonful glycerine and one teaspoonful of cider vinegar. Apply after shampooing and rinsing, and leave on for fifteen minutes. Rinse well. You will find other suggestions for natural hair care products you can prepare yourself included in Chapter 11.

A CHANGE OF COLOUR

Many women (and men) succumb to the temptation to change the natural shade of their hair, despite the effort involved, and with little regard for the current evidence which suggests that hair dyes may be linked with cancer. The government in this country is keeping a close watch on these products, while in America they now carry a cancer-risk warning.

Alternatives in the natural field are limited, and are likely to produce a less dramatic effect, but they are safe. Most need to be used repeatedly over a period of time before there is any marked difference in hair colour. Test any hair dye on the ends of your hair before applying it to your head (the ends are more porous than the rest of the hair, and enable you to see the result before it is too late).

Herbs have been used for many centuries as colouring agents, the most common being sage for dark or greying hair, and chamomile for fair hair. To use herbs as colourants, make them into a rinse and apply after shampooing. For instance, to lighten brown hair, add 2-4 tablespoonsful of chamomile flowers to a pint (550ml) of boiling water and stand for up to three hours. Strain, and use the resulting liquid to rinse the hair several times, holding a basin under your head to catch the liquid so that you can re-use it.

An alternative which is more effective, although also more trouble, is to make your own herbal hair dye. This is produced by taking four tablespoonsful of the herb of your choice and leaving them to stand in a cupful of boiling water for at least twenty minutes. Strain and mix the liquid to a paste with kaolin (a fine clay powder available from chemists). Apply this mixture to the roots of your hair, and them comb it through. Leave on for between twenty minutes and one hour, depending on the desired effect – the longer you leave it, the more marked will be the change.

One effective natural hair colourant which can be purchased ready-made is henna. This imparts a reddish tinge to dark hair, without changing the chemical structure of the hair as other dyes do. Instead it coats the hair and gives it extra body – in fact, henna is often used as a hair conditioner. Henna preparations can be bought in some health food shops and chemists, but follow the instructions carefully or you may find the results rather unpredictable.

YOUR HAIR CARE CHART

Hair Type	How to Recognize It	Shampooing	Special Care
Normal	Shiny without being greasy. Fairly easy to manage. Looks good for about a week after shampooing.	Wash once a week following general instructions. Use a conditioner every other week.	Massage daily. Use a protein conditioner twice a month.
Greasy	Looks good for a day or two, but quickly becomes lank.	Wash as little as possible, at the most twice a week. Pay particular attention to massaging shampoo in. Rinse thoroughly, adding cider vinegar or lemon juice to rinse water.	Massage daily. Use a dry shampoo like bran or oatmeal. Use a protein conditioner once a month.
Dry	Difficult to control. Looks dull with dry ends. Scalp often feels itchy.	Wash once a week using a cream shampoo. Use a conditioner each time.	Massage dialy. Use an oil treatment once a fortnight.

CHAPTER SEVEN

A PAIR OF SPARKLING EYES

It takes only a poor night's sleep, a bout of crying, or a heavy cold to make your eyes look dull, red and strained – hardly conducive to beauty, you must admit. Clear white sparkling eyes are an essential part of looking beautiful, but the eyes are even more directly affected by external factors than the skin and hair.

VITAMIN A

The first requisite for beautiful eyes is a good diet which supplies plenty of vitamin A. This vitamin is closely connected with good eyesight and clear eyes, and especially with the ability to see in dim light or the dark. Foods rich in vitamin A include butter and margarine, oily fish, and orange and yellow fruits and vegetables. Other vitamins essential to good eyesight are vitamins B2, C and D. Where there is a lack of vitamin B2, eyes often become bloodshot, itchy and watery.

Vitamin A is especially important to those who use their eyes a lot (e.g. reading, typing, etc.), since these people use up extra vitamin A. Equally important is to see that you work in plenty of light, which should come from above, behind or the side, but not from the front since this tends to make you squint, thus encouraging wrinkles as well as poor eyesight.

If you use your eyes a lot, try to rest them at intervals during the day. This can be done by palming, which simply means covering both eyes with the palms of your hands so that all light is excluded. Keep your eyes covered, but open, for five minutes.

EYE EXERCISES

Eye exercises are quick and easy to do and are worth

the effort since they help the eyesight by strengthening the muscles, while at the same time reducing eye strain. A good exercise is to roll your eyes round in circles while keeping your head still. Rotate the eyes in each direction, trying to do this twelve times a day. Another simple but effective exercise is to hold your index finger about three inches from your face. Look at it closely, and then quickly extend your arm as far as it will go in front of you, all the time following your finger with your eyes. Then bring your finger back to within a few inches of your face. Repeat this several times.

HELP FOR RED, PUFFY EYES

Refresh tired, reddened eyes by placing a slice of cucumber over the closed lids while you rest with your feet up. You'll find this very cooling and refreshing. Tea bags, too, can be used for the same purpose – but wring them out first!

Bathe tired, strained eyes with an eye bath made from the herb eyebright, used for centuries for this purpose and still included in many of today's commercial eyewashes. Prepare the lotion by pouring a cupful of boiling water over one teaspoon of the dried herb and leave until cool. Strain and use the liquid to bathe the eyes.

Dark circles and swelling under the eyes can be caused by lack of sleep, which is another good reason for getting plenty of it. Eight hours a night is the ideal amount for most people, so when you are out late, try and make up for those lost hours the following night. Reduce swelling or bags under the eyes by applying ice-cold witch hazel, water or milk. Dab this on with cotton wool.

Puffiness around the eyes can also be caused by applying the wrong sort of cosmetics. The skin around the eyes is very thin and delicate, containing no sebaceous glands and with little circulation. This means it needs extra care. Never use astringents, heavy creams, or face masks around the eyes, since these will stretch the skin leading to puffiness and premature wrinkles.

Many women find that they are allergic to a particular brand of eye make up, even after using it for a number of years. If you develop sore red eyes all of a sudden, stop using any make up for a few days and see if the condition clears up. If it does, then it is worth trying another cosmetic brand, such as one of the hypo-allergenic ranges which are produced for those with sensitive skin. If the condition persists even without the use of make up, you should see your doctor without delay.

USING A MOISTURISER

Regular moisturising is as important for the eye area as it is for the rest of the face, since it helps to soften and lubricate the skin and to delay the formation of wrinkles. However, you need to choose your moisturiser with care, opting for a special eye cream which is very light in texture. Many people have found that an eye cream is more effective if it contains vitamin E – buy a product containing this, or add the contents of a capsule to your eye cream. There's a recipe for vitamin E eye cream on page 82.

Unless you apply your eye cream correctly you will be doing your eyes more harm than good. Here's the right way to apply cream to the eye area: using the pad of your forefinger, start at the inner corner of the eye and very gently spread the cream over the eyelid to the outer corner, then back under the eye to the centure. You should also use this method when applying any kind of eye make up, and when removing it too.

REMOVING EYE MAKE UP

As far as this is concerned, always use a remover designed specifically for the eyes. While other lotions may effectively remove the make up, many will also make the eyes red and sore. Make it a habit to remove eye make up every night without fail. It may be the last thing you feel like doing when you are tired, but it is worth the effort or your neglect will show in spots, and sparse, weakened eyelashes.

When removing eye make up, rub the cotton wool or remover pad gently down over the eyelid and upper lashes, then open the eyes and wipe the lower lashes, working towards the inner corner of the eye as described above. Make sure you remove all traces of the remover, since most of these tend to be greasy, and could cause whiteheads if left on the skin.

STEP BY STEP EYE MAKE UP

Eye make up, if skilfully applied, can considerably improve or alter a woman's appearance. It can be used, for instance, to disguise the fact that your eyes are too deep set, or too wide apart. On the other hand, eye make up incorrectly used can quite spoil the look of someone who would otherwise be beautiful. If you want to wear eye make up regularly, it might well be worth investing in a visit to a beauty salon, where you can pick up invaluable tips on the right way to go about things.

EYE SHADOW

The first step is to apply your eye shadow in whatever form you choose – powder, cream or stick. If your eyelids are at all dry, you will find that a powder shadow stays put longer than other kinds. Remember that bright shades of shadow serve to emphasize the eyes, while deeper tones de-emphasize. The easiest way to apply eye shadow is to use a special eye make up brush, which gives you more control over application.

EYELINER

Use of an eyeliner should be restricted to a shade which is close to that of your eyes, so that you can make a soft line rather than a dark heavy one, which is most unflattering. Liquid and cake liners both give a fairly sharp line, while a pencil is more subtle. After applying the liner, smudge it gently with your finger tip to blend it into the lashes and the shadow. Most eye shapes are improved by a thin line from the centre of the lid, very close to the lashes, to the outer corner of the eye, making the line slightly thicker as you go.

MASCARA

Next comes the mascara, which should be applied in several thin coats to prevent clogging the lashes. Coat both the top and bottom of the upper lashes, brushing down from the top and then upwards. Use downward strokes for the lower lashes, and allow each coat to dry before applying another. If your lashes are out of condition, use a non-waterproof cake mascara which is easier to remove and less harmful to the eyes. To thicken your lashes, an application of talcum powder or face powder in between coats of mascara is very effective. After the final coat of mascara, use a dry brush to gently separate the lashes.

PLUCKING THE EYEBROWS

This should be done without altering the basic shape of the face, and for this reason you should only remove hairs from below the eyebrows and from each end. When correctly shaped, the brows should start above the inner corner of the eye, with the highest part of the curve above the outer rim of the iris, and ending at the point where a diagonal line drawn from the nose to the outer corner of the eye would cross the brow.

The best time for plucking the eyebrows is after a bath, while your skin is still warm, to minimize any redness or soreness. Always pull the hairs out in the direction in which they grow. Finish up by dabbing a little mild toner on to the plucked area to discourage any redness.

CHAPTER EIGHT

LOOKING AFTER YOUR TEETH

Did you know that 37 per cent of adults in the U.K. over the age of sixteen have none of their own teeth? It is a staggering statistic, and unless you take proper care of your teeth, you could be well on the way to acquiring a set of dentures yourself. Both dental decay, and the gum disease which often accompanies it, are preventable with the proper care.

Dental care should begin as early in life as possible, and almost as soon as a child acquires his first teeth he should be encouraged to brush them regularly. He won't yet understand what it is all about, but it will get him into the habit, and if you choose one of the toothpastes especially made for babies he will enjoy the occasion too.

HOW TO CLEAN YOUR TEETH

Most people know that teeth should be brushed after every meal (even if they don't do so), but not so many realize that there is a right and a wrong way to clean your teeth. First of all, you must choose the right toothbrush, the best being a firm, densely tufted, natural bristle one. If your brush is too hard it may irritate the gums and cause unnecessary bleeding, while if it is too soft it will not do an effiicient job of cleaning. Your brush should be replaced every three or four months. Use a toothpaste without harsh abrasives which may damage the tooth enamel, and without chemical bleaching agents or synthetic colourings. There are a couple of natural toothpastes on sale in health food shops, or a good homemade one can be produced by mixing equal quantities of bicarbonate of soda and salt.

The way to brush your teeth is with an up and down movement, not from side to side. Brush the upper teeth downwards, and the lower teeth upwards. Start with the back teeth, and be sure to brush both their fronts and backs. Now brush the middle teeth, finishing up with the front teeth. Don't be afraid to touch your gums with the brush, since they benefit from gentle stimulation to improve the circulation.

A quick brush is a waste of time because although your teeth may appear clean, they will still be coated with an invisible layer of plaque. And it is the presence of plaque which causes tooth decay. The whole brushing procedure should take you three minutes to perform. If you are unsure whether you are getting your teeth really clean, invest in a packet of disclosing tablets. These contain a harmless dye which colours any remaining dirt or plaque a vivid red so that there is no mistaking where you have omitted to clean.

Plaque, by the way, is a mixture of bacteria, saliva and food residues which is responsible for both tooth decay and gum disease. Plaque must be removed daily, since if left for more than twenty-four hours it produces acids which attack the enamel and start the decay. It also causes gum inflammation and bleeding, which are early warning signals of gum disease. Because plaque is invisible it can be present on even the whitest of teeth, and with normal brushing you can still miss 80 per cent of the plaque.

Just as important as regular and thorough brushing of your teeth, is to make frequent visits to your dentist. Most people have a dread of the dentist, imagining that they will be subjected to all sorts of excruciating torture, but with the modern methods of today, dental treatment is rarely painful. You certainly should not put off going to the dentist, and should make it a habit to visit him every six months for a check up. A dentist will also be able to give you any advice you may need on cosmetic problems, such as crooked or chipped teeth.

Bad breath is as unpleasant and embarrassing for the sufferer as it is for those he comes into contact with. If your digestion is functioning efficiently you are unlikely to suffer from bad breath – unless, of course, you have just indulged in a highly seasoned meal or a portion of garlic bread! Freshen your breath naturally by chewing fresh parsley or watercress, or by using rosewater or lavender water as a mouth wash.

DIET AND YOUR TEETH

Diet has a part to play in dental health, and it is thanks to all the refined sugary foods that most people eat in such quantity that we are witnessing an increase in dental decay. These foods form a sticky deposit on the teeth, producing an ideal breeding ground for the bacteria which cause decay.

Try to cut white sugar and foods containing it right out of your diet, and restrict your sugar intake in all forms. Make sure your diet includes plenty of crisp, crunchy foods like raw vegetables, hard biscuits, or crunchy wholemeal bread. When your children begin to teethe, chewing on a stale bread crust, a stick of raw carrot, or even a cooked chicken bone, eases any tenderness and irritation.

The person who eats a wholefood diet will have less likelihood of dental decay simply because the foods eaten are healthier. At the same time, unrefined foods leave larger particles in the mouth, which take the enzymes longer to break down. The ideal way to end a meal is with fresh fruit like an apple, which helps to remove any sticky deposits, especially from the back teeth where decay is most common. Also good for cleaning the teeth is to munch on a stick of raw celery or carrot. Sweetened drinks like fruit squashes and fizzy drinks should be replaced with natural unsweetened juices or milk.

Children should be discouraged at an early age

from eating too many sweets. Offer them fresh fruit, raw celery or carrot, nuts or dried fruits as alternatives. Obviously it is impossible to prevent a child from eating any sweets, especially once he starts school, but it helps if you explain to him the reasons why sweet eating is bad (i.e., for teeth and health), and the importance of brushing his teeth afterwards. See if he will limit his sweet eating to the end of a meal, after which he can brush his teeth before bacteria have a chance to form.

The nutrients your diet needs to contain for strong healthy teeth are the minerals phosphorous and calcium, vitamins A and D, and protein. Vitamin C is essential for healthy gums, and bleeding in this area is often one of the first signs of a vitamin C deficiency.

If you are in the habit of drinking strong tea or coffee, or of smoking cigarettes, your teeth are likely to become yellow and discoloured. Since these practices are bad for your health too, it's worth trying to give them up. However, if all else fails, scrubbing the teeth with lemon peel helps to remove any stains. It is important to rinse your mouth out well after using this, otherwise you create an unnaturally acid medium. A powder for stain removal can be made by mixing three tablespoonsful of bicarbonate of soda and two tablespoonsful of salt. Rub the teeth well with this mixture.

CHAPTER NINE

CARING FOR YOUR HANDS AND FEET

Your hands have a hard life. Not only are they exposed to all kinds of weather conditions, but they are constantly being immersed in water which contains such powerful chemical solutions as washing powder, bleach, washing up liquid, etc. It is little wonder, therefore, that your hands are one of the first parts of the body to show signs of neglect and ageing.

However careful you may be to keep them hidden from view, people tend to notice the state of your hands. That is one good reason for taking care of them; another is that, as with most things, preventing trouble is considerably easier than curing it.

WEAR GLOVES
Rule number one is to protect your hands in such a way that they do not come into direct contact with a constant barrage of chemicals. This means wearing a pair of rubber gloves for all household chores like washing, washing up, and cleaning. They may make you feel ham-fisted, but if you choose a pair of fine rubber gloves you will find that you soon get used to wearing them. And for jobs where your hands will not be immersed in water, cotton gloves can be worn. Keep a pair of rubber gloves in a prominent place next to the sink so that you have no excuse for forgetting to wear them.

MOISTURE
Equally important to the state of your hands is plenty of moisture. However religiously you may wear your gloves, your hands are still going to be immersed in

water frequently (e.g., when bathing or washing yourself), and this tends to dry out the natural oils. The way to counteract this is to apply a nourishing cream every time your hands have been in water, or after every rough job. Once again, a jar or bottle of handcream strategically placed in the kitchen and bathroom will act as a constant reminder. A nourishing lotion you can easily make yourself is half a cup of glycerine mixed with a cup of rosewater. Variations to this basic recipe can be made by adding two tablespoonsful of lemon juice, or by heating two tablespoonsful of glycerine, and adding two tablespoonsful of cornflour and a cupful of rosewater. Other handcream recipes for you to make at home can be found in Chapter 11).

Your hands will also benefit if you replace over-alkaline soaps with glycerine or vegetable-based ones which are less drying. Rinsing your hands in cider vinegar after washing helps to restore the skin's natural acid coating. Always ensure that you dry your hands thoroughly after washing.

If you suffer from poor circulation (suggested by constantly cold hands with a blotchy bluish tinge) always wear warm gloves when you go out in winter, and carefully massage your hands with long stroking movements whenever you apply hand cream. Typing, playing the piano, or exercises like strumming the fingers on a table all help improve circulation. Chilblains benefit from the same treatment, but also ensure that your diet contains ample calcium.

TREATING NEGLECTED HANDS

If your hands have been neglected long enough to get into a very poor state, start by using a well-soaped pumice stone to rub off any roughened skin. Then soak your hands in a mixture of equal parts of salt, Epsom salts and water softener, dissolved in warm water. If you let your hands soak in this mixture for a few minutes you will open the pores and stimulate the circulation, after which you can rub in a rich hand cream. Repeat this soaking and moisturising procedure every day until your hands get back to their normal shape.

Treat your hands once or twice a week to a massage with a really rich cream. Once a week precede this by soaking your hands in warmed oil (preferably olive or almond) for between five to thirty minutes. This is a great treatment for dry hands and nails.

Whenever you are using a lemon in the kitchen, keep the skin and pulp and rub this over your hands to whiten and soften them, and to clean your nails and cuticles.

CARE FOR FINGER NAILS

Nails are formed by very tightly packed layers of skin cells which grow from the dermis skin layer. Only half the nail is visible, the other half (known as the matrix) is also oval in shape and extends to the first finger joint. Nails are composed of keratin (as is the hair) which is formed mainly from protein and calcium. That is why a diet rich in these two nutrients is an essential part of healthy nails. Other important nutrients are iron, potassium, iodine and the B vitamins. Split or hang nails, ridges, white spots or flaking nails are all signs of a faulty diet.

The finger nails, like the hands, have to pay the price for being constantly subjected to abuse, so any hand care programme should incorporate the nails. Give your nails a regular manicure once a week. Always use an emery board which is less harsh than a metal file, to shape your nails. File in one direction only, from the sides to the centre, since a sawing motion will cause flaking. Nails should be filed round, rather than pointed, although if your nails are short and inclined to break and flake, filing them square helps them to grow evenly.

Clean under the nails with an orange stick tipped with cotton wool. An orange stick should also be used to gently shape the cuticles, to avoid breaking or tearing the skin. The best time to shape the cuticles is after your hands have been in water (e.g., after a bath) since this helps to soften the skin ready for shaping. Otherwise, you can soak your fingers in warm water and herbal shampoo before your manicure. Nails and cuticles also benefit from a cuticle cream to keep them in good condition. Make your own by mixing two tablespoonsful of petroleum jelly with half a teaspoonful of glycerine. Massage this in well.

Avoid wearing nail varnish whenever possible, since this has a drying effect on the nails. If you do wear it, apply a base coat first to protect the nails. The worst offenders are the pearlized nail polishes (did you know they contain fish scales?) which are more drying than the cream ones. Always remove nail polish at least once a week, since an accumulation of several coats of polish can make nails even more dry and flaky. Nail varnish remover also tends to be very drying, so counteract this by adding a teaspoonful of glycerine to a bottle of acetone. This also has the advantage of being considerably cheaper than proprietary brands of remover.

You will probably find that the condition of your nails improves during the summer, this being due to better circulation. You can also improve the circulation by buffing the nails, since this stimulates the flow of blood around the nails. Buffing is done with a specially designed pad covered in leather (available from many chemists). When using this, always buff in one direction.

Drinking cider vinegar each day is said to help strengthen nails, as well as being good for your general health. Take a tablespoonful of the vinegar in a glass of water three times a day before meals.

DON'T FORGET YOUR FEET
With feet, it is often a case of out of sight, out of

mind. Because they are hidden away for much of the time, it is easy to forget about looking after them. But feet need regular care not only to make them look good, but to avoid such crippling conditions as corns and callouses, which can turn even a quick trip round the shops into a painful feat(!) of endurance. If conditions like this develop, it is a good idea to consult a chiropodist.

Ill-fitting shoes are the most likely cause of foot problems, so always choose shoes for comfort rather than fashion. Shoes should support the arch of the foot well, and should allow ample room for the toes.

Keep your feet in good shape with a few simple exercises. First thing in the morning, arch your ankles, bend your toes and flex the whole foot. Walking is one of the best beauty treatments (provided your shoes fit well), while standing on tiptoe is a good exercise and can be practised at odd moments throughout the day.

For feet that are sore and swollen after a long day, relax with your feet higher than your head, and gently massage your legs and feet. Soak your feet in cold water and cider vinegar, in salt water, or in warm water containing a handful of nettle leaves. Cold feet respond well to a massage with olive oil, while an old remedy for tired feet is alternate soaking in hot and cold water, ending with the cold.

Once a week at bathtime give your feet a good going over. While your skin is still warm from the bath, rub off any hard skin with a pumice stone. Then trim the nails, cutting and filing as necessary, but following the general advice given for finger nails. Unlike the finger nails, toe nails should be shaped straight across. If rounded or pointed they can cause discomfort or give rise to ingrowing nails. After shaping, massage in a cuticle cream and shape the cuticles with an orange stick.

Clean well around the nails with an orange stick tipped with cotton wool, paying particular attention to the sides of the nails where dirt tends to collect.

After this pedicure, rub plenty of moisturising body lotion all over your feet.

To keep your feet smelling fresh, especially in hot weather, apply a deodorising talcum powder each morning after washing. Always wash socks or tights daily or, better still, go without if the weather permits.

CHAPTER TEN

HOW TO HAVE A BEAUTIFUL HOLIDAY

As you pack your holiday suitcase, beauty is probably far from your thoughts. After all, the last thing you want to be bothered with while you are away is routine of any sort, including a beauty routine. All the same it is worth sparing a thought before you leave home for a few items which will help you keep up a good appearance while you're away – there is no point in undoing all that good work you've been doing at home!

You may enjoy soaking up the sun, and a deep golden sun tan may do wonders for your looks and your morale, but too much sun is bad for you. It has a drying and ageing effect on the skin and, according to some authorities, even causes skin cancer. This is not to say that you need spend all summer sitting in the shade, but you do need to take extra care of your skin if you are going to bask in the sunshine.

You will probably know from bitter experience just how much or how little sun your body can take. The colour of your hair and skin is a good indication, those with a dark complexion being able to tolerate much more sun than the fair-skinned. How easily you tan is determined by a pigment called melanin – dark-skinned people have a lot of it, fair haired people have less, and red heads have virtually none.

When the skin is exposed to the ultra-violet rays of the sun, the skin cells are stimulated to increase the production of melanin in order to protect the skin from burning. It is when you have too little melanin, or when it is produced too slowly, that you experience the agonies of sunburn.

SUCCESSFUL SUNTANNING
Whatever your skin type, the secret of a successful
tan lies in taking it very easy at first. And – rather than
ruin a long-awaited holiday through suffering
sunburn – choose a really good suntanning cream.
Most sun creams work on the principle of screening
out the stronger of the sun's ultra violet rays, but
allowing some through. This gives your skin a chance
to build up its own protection without you getting
burned. A few sun creams block out all the burning
rays, and these are the ones to choose if you have a
very sensitive skin.

If you have a dry skin which burns easily, it is best
to use a cream or oil which will serve to moisturise
your skin while also protecting it. Sunbathe for very
short periods at first, gradually building up the
length of time as the days go by. You have got to be
patient if you want a tan which is not patchy or
peeling.

A normal skin can use any of the suntanning
preparations, whether it be oil, cream or lotion. An
oily skin, though, would do better with a light lotion.
This is one time when a greasy skin comes into its
own – it is likely to tan faster and become less
dehydrated than other skin types. If you are prone to
spots, you will also find that these improve after
exposure to the sun.

HOME-MADE SUN LOTIONS
There is a bewildering choice of products on sale for
promoting suntans or for preventing sunburn. If you
don't know which one to go for, you may prefer to
make your own – and save yourself a few pounds at
the same time. Sesame seed oil can be used on its
own, or can be mixed with other ingredients. This oil
penetrates and softens the skin, and of all the oils is
the one which absorbs the ultra-violet rays most
fully. Try mixing a cup of sesame or olive oil with half
a cupful of cider vinegar, a teaspoonful of iodine,

and a few drops of lavender oil (the inclusion of the latter ingredient not only improves the scent but also helps to keep insects away). A mixture of two thirds sunflower oil to one third of lemon juice or cider vinegar is used in many countries as a sun tan lotion. There is another recipe on page 82.

Whatever suntanning product you choose, remember to apply it every couple of hours while you are sunbathing, and after swimming. Pay particular attention to your nose, shoulders, chest, the lower part of your stomach, and the tops of your legs. These are all danger areas which need extra applications of suncream to prevent burning.

Vitamin A is said to help prevent sunburn by building up the skin's own resistance more quickly than normal. Take extra vitamin A both before and during your holiday. While the level of vitamin A in the blood drops after intensive exposure to ultra violet rays, the production of vitamin D is encouraged. In sunnier climates than our own, the action of sunlight on the skin is often a major source of vitamin D, which is poorly distributed in foods. Sunbathing also depletes vitamin B levels, since these nutrients are involved in the production of melanin, so remember to pack your brewer's yeast tablets.

REPLACING LOST MOISTURE

Because the sun has such a drying effect on the skin, it is essential to counteract this by applying lashings of moisturiser. Otherwise you may end up looking wrinkled and leathery – hardly the desired effect! You just cannot apply too much moisture while you are in the sun, even if your skin tends to be naturally greasy.

Make it a habit to moisturise your body all over every evening while on holiday, and add an oil to your bath water too. Each morning rub coconut oil all over yourself, and then wash it off in the shower or bath. Salt water aggravates the dryness, and should be washed off with fresh water as soon as possible, or at least every evening. When you return home, and your tan begins to fade along with your holiday memories, don't leave off the moisturising treatment. It helps to preserve your tan by slowing up the natural shedding of the outer layers of skin, and discourages any peeling or flakiness.

If you do overdo the sunbathing and find yourself suffering the agonies of sunburn, an application of cider vinegar and water, of mashed cucumber, strong tea or milk helps to soothe the burn.

LOOKING AFTER YOUR HAIR

It is not just your skin which is likely to suffer on a sunny holiday. Salt water, sea breezes and sun also combine to play havoc with your hair. Always wash the salt water out at the end of the day, and wear a protective head-covering if the sun is very hot. This is particularly important if your hair is dyed or bleached, since the sun can often change the colour dramatically. Choose a rich cream shampoo, and follow this with a conditioner to put back the oils the sun has taken out. Even greasy hair will benefit from conditioning while you are on holiday.

IN COLDER CLIMATES

On a cold weather holiday, extra moisture and protection are again important, since the skin suffers from either extreme of temperature. Especially likely to suffer from the cold are dry or sensitive skins. Whatever your skin type, apply a rich moisturiser and a light foundation before venturing out into the cold. These will protect your face from the elements, help prevent thread veins and an unsightly red nose. Apply a lip salve to stop your lips becoming sore and chapped, and use a rich hand cream and warm gloves to protect your hands. In the evenings after a day spent out in the cold, have a relaxing warm bath, followed by an all-over application of body lotion.

HOLIDAY BEAUTY CHECK LIST

Hot Weather Holiday	Cold Weather Holiday
Suntanning preparation	Rich moisturiser
Sunburn soother (just in case)	Light foundation cream
Moisturiser	Lip salve
Body Lotion	Body Lotion
Bath oil	Rich hand cream
Coconut oil	Warm gloves
Headcovering	
Brewer's yeast tablets	
Vitamin A supplement	
Rich cream shampoo	
Hair conditioner	

CHAPTER ELEVEN

HOME-MADE COSMETICS

Because cosmetics do not by law have to declare a list of ingredients, there is usually no way of telling just what has gone into a particular product. This means that some of the ingredients of the cosmetics you buy could, for all you know, be doing your skin more harm than good. This problem occurs particularly with those who are allergic to certain substances, and who have no way of knowing whether the offending ingredient is present in a given product.

One way to be sure of just what you are putting on your skin is to make your own cosmetics. It is an idea which will appeal to any do-it-yourself enthusiast or keen cook, but you don't need to be an expert in either of these fields to obtain enjoyment and success from making your own skin care products. As you will see from the suggestions later in this chapter, some of the ideas are so simple that a child could make them, and even the more complicated recipes are easily mastered if you follow the instructions through step by step.

Another plus point for home-made cosmetics is their cost. Those women for whom expensive cosmetics are out of reach have no excuse for neglecting their skin when so many household items can benefit the complexion. No expensive equipment is needed, and the few special ingredients you will have to buy are unlikely to break the bank, especially since they are used in very small quantities and so last a long time.

There is no point in making up gallons of a lotion or cream at one session. For one thing, unless you have tried a particular recipe before, you may find that it does not suit your particular skin. Since home-made cosmetics are made from fresh ingredients and without preservatives they also have a shorter life than bought products. If stored in airtight containers most cosmetics will keep for a month or two, by which time you have probably used them up anyway. However, a recipe containing any ingredients you would normally store in the refrigerator is best refrigerated. One of the advantages of making up small batches at a time is that you can afford to experiment with all sorts of different cosmetics – an experiment which would set you back a lot of money if you used shop products.

You should be able to obtain any of the special items mentioned in the following recipes from your chemist. However, in case of difficulty, John Bell and Croydon of Wigmore Street, London W1, should be able to help. Many recipes call for lanolin, which comes in two forms: either hydrous or anhydrous. The difference is that the anhydrous lanolin has no added water, while the hydrous has a high water content. The following recipes use anhydrous lanolin. The kind of oil you use in your cosmetics is governed by the type of skin you have. If your skin is greasy you are best advised to use mineral oil rather than vegetable oil, since this is less penetrating. For those with dry or normal skins, any kind of vegetable oil is suitable. Most of the recipes given here do not include any perfume, but if you want a more fragrant cosmetic, try adding a few drops of an essential oil such as lavender oil. These can be obtained from Baldwins, of 77 Walworth Road, London SE17.

COSMETICS FROM THE KITCHEN CUPBOARD

You may be surprised to learn that many of the ingredients you would normally have in your kitchen can also be used as natural beauty aids. To get yourself attuned to making your own cosmetics, start off by trying some of these simple ideas using household ingredients.

CIDER VINEGAR

Mixed with equal parts of water, this cleanses and tones the skin. If added to the final rinse water when washing the hair, it also helps eliminate dandruff and restores the hair's natural acid coating, which is usually removed by the shampoo. A cupful of cider vinegar in the bathwater is said to relieve aches and pains, while drinking a tablespoonful of cider vinegar in water three times a day before meals helps to strengthen finger nails.

CUCUMBER JUICE

This makes a good toner, or you can mash whole cucumber and use it as a toning face mask. Obtain cucumber juice by liquidising and straining a chopped cucumber, or mash and sieve the cucumber. Cucumber does not keep well, so any product containing it should be stored under refrigeration. Slices of cucumber placed over the eyes while you relax for 15 minutes help to refresh and soothe tired eyes.

EGG WHITE

Beaten and applied to a greasy skin as a face mask, egg white helps to refine large pores and tone the skin. To vary, add the juice of half a lemon.

EGG YOLK

Mixed with a tablespoonful of vegetable oil, this makes a good face mask for dry or sensitive skins. Make it more nourishing by adding a tablespoonful of honey. See page 52 for an egg yolk shampoo, or try the following: mix 1 egg with 1 to 2 tablespoonsful of herbal shampoo. Beat in a tablespoonful of gelatine for extra conditioning. Make a hair conditioner by beating together 3 egg yolks, and a few drops each of glycerine, cider vinegar and vegetable oil. Gently warm the mixture and apply it to your hair half an hour before shampooing.

HONEY

This can be used on its own as a face mask for dry or normal skins. When combined with oatmeal it helps refine a greasy skin. To make a honey hair conditioner, beat one egg with a teaspoonful of honey and two teaspoonsful of vegetable oil. Massage into your hair, and leave on for half an hour before shampooing.

LEMON JUICE

Lemon juice mixed with an equal quantity of water or rosewater tones and bleaches the skin. Add it to the final rinse water when shampooing your hair, or comb or spray on undiluted juice as a hair setting lotion.

OATMEAL

Mixed with honey, milk or water, oatmeal makes a good cleansing and refining face mask. Oatmeal and/or bran can be used as a dry shampoo, by rubbing well into the hair and then brushing out thoroughly. For a cleansing, soothing bath, tie a tablespoonful of bran or oatmeal in a piece of muslin or cheesecloth and place in the bathwater. Make a paste for washing with by combining a tablespoonful each of oatmeal, dried and ground orange peel, and ground almonds. Add enough water to give a paste.

POTATOES

Grated raw and applied to the eye area, they help eliminate puffiness and bags.

SEA SALT

Sea salt dissolved in ice cold water or applied direct to the wet skin refines open pores and helps to remove the surface layer of dead skin.

YOGURT

This makes a good cleanser for oily skins. It also helps to improve unmanageable hair if massaged well in for about three minutes after shampooing. Rinse out thoroughly.

APPLES
Use as the basis for a dry skin face mask, or a hand lotion. Finely chop and mash an apple, then add half a teaspoonful of milk and a tablespoonful of honey.

BREWER'S YEAST POWDER
Used as an ingredient in a facial, this is good for the circulation. Don't use it more than once a week, and apply a thin coating of oil to the skin first. Because this mask can bring out impurities, avoid using it before going out anywhere special. Dissolve half a teaspoonful of yeast in a little water, and add a tablespoonful of honey, a tablespoonful of vegetable oil, and half a teaspoonful of cider vinegar. Mix well. If your skin is greasy, add a tablespoonful of yogurt, buttermilk or whipped egg white. For dry skins, add a tablespoonful of sour cream and one beaten egg yolk.

GELATINE
This helps to set hair if added to final rinse water. Dissolve two tablespoonsful in two cups of boiling water before adding.

ROSEWATER AND WITCHHAZEL
These can be combined to make a simple toner. Use equal quantities for a greasy skin, or 3/4 rosewater to 1/4 witchazel for normal skin. If your skin is very dry, dilute the toner with a little water.

SOME SIMPLE COSMETIC RECIPES

CUCUMBER AND MINT TONING LOTION
½ cucumber
2 tablespoonsful witchazel
4 tablespoonsful mint leaves
1 tablespoonful rosewater

Put all the ingredients into a liquidizer and blend until smooth. Store in a refrigerator.

SUMMER TONER WITH RASPBERRIES
2 cupsful raspberries
a teaspoonful honey
1 cupful rose petals
2 pt. (1¼l) cider vinegar

Steep the raspberries and rose petals in the cider vinegar and honey for a month. Strain and add an equal quantity of water.

ROSE CLEANSING CREAM
2 teaspoonsful castile soap,
   grated
4 tablespoonsful lanolin
2 tablespoonsful oil
2 tablespoonsful rosewater
Pinch of borax (if needed)

Melt the soap with the oil and lanolin in a double boiler (a bowl over a pan of boiling water will do). Add the rosewater a little at a time, beating with a whisk. Remove from the heat and whisk until cool. If the mixture separates, whisk again adding the borax. Pot and leave in the refrigerator to set.

CUCUMBER CLEANSER
3 teaspoonsful beeswax
5 teaspoonsful mineral oil
1 teaspoonful glycerine
4 tablespoonsful vegetable oil
4 tablespoonsful cucumber juice
Pinch of borax

Melt the oils and wax over hot water. Gently heat the rest of the ingredients together until the borax has dissolved. Add the borax mixture to the oils a drop at a time, stirring constantly. Beat until cool. Refrigerate.

HONEY MOISTURISER

3 tablespoonsful lanolin
4 tablespoonsful warm water
$\frac{1}{2}$ tablespoonful honey

Melt the lanolin over hot water. Slowly add the honey and water, beating well. Remove from the heat and beat until cool. Do not refrigerate, or the cream may separate.

LEMON NOURISHING CREAM

2 eggs
1 teaspoonful lemon juice
2 beaten egg yolks
1 teaspoonful glycerine
2 teaspoonsful vegetable oil
2 tablespoonsful water

Blend the eggs, glycerine and lemon juice. Slowly add enough oil to give a thick cream. Add the egg yolks and water a little at a time, stirring constantly. Refrigerate.

LIME BODY LOTION

3 tablespoonsful rosewater
2 tablespoonsful lime juice
1 tablespoonful glycerine

Blend all the ingredients together. Use after a bath. This lotion is excellent for dry skin, and has the advantage of not being too oily.

BUBBLE BATH

1 egg
1 teaspoonful gelatine
$\frac{1}{2}$ cupful herbal shampoo

Mix all the ingredients together with an electric whisk. Add to the bath water under the running tap.

ALMOND HAND CREAM
$\frac{1}{2}$ oz. (12g) white wax
2 fl.oz. (50ml) rosewater
6 tablespoonsful almond oil
1 teaspoonful vegetable oil

Melt the wax and oils over hot water. Beat in the rosewater drop by drop, and continue beating until the mixture cools.

MILK LOTION FOR ROUGH SKIN
$\frac{1}{2}$ pt. (275ml) milk
$\frac{1}{2}$ oz. (12g) bicarbonate of soda
$\frac{1}{2}$ oz. (12g) glycerine
$\frac{1}{2}$ oz. (12g) borax

Warm the milk and slowly add the other ingredients. Heat gently until the borax dissolves.

VITAMIN E EYE CREAM
1 tablespoonful lanolin
2 teaspoonsful cold water
$1\frac{1}{2}$ tablespoonsful almond oil
1 vitamin E capsule

Melt the lanolin and oil over hot water. Remove from the heat and add the water and the contents of the vitamin E capsule. Beat well with an electric mixer or wooden spoon. This gives quite a runny cream.

SUNTAN LOTION
4 tablespoonsful lanolin
2 tablespoonsful almond oil
3 tablespoonsful sesame oil
$\frac{1}{2}$ cupful strong tea

Melt the oils and lanolin over hot water. Remove from the heat and beat in the strained tea, using a wooden spoon or electric mixer. The tannin in the tea acts as a natural sun screen.

INDEX

INDEX

Other recommended books

KELP FOR BETTER HEALTH AND VITALITY

NOURISHING FOOD FROM SEAWEED

Frank Wilson. Explains the nutritional and medicinal benefits of kelp and other seaweeds. There are some 800 varieties around the shores of the British Isles alone, most of them representing a substantial nutritional resource. Kelp in particular contains a wide range of essential vitamins, minerals and trace elements. In Wales, Ireland and Scotland seaweed was a traditional food; in Europe it was utilized as fertilizer, potash and iodine. Unusual recipes include: Sprout and Seaweed soup; Kombu fry; Dulse and Fruit salad.

HERBAL TEAS FOR HEALTH AND HEALING

Ceres. *Illustrated.* Over a hundred tea-making herbs are described in this delightful book. Some are slightly stimulating, others are tonics for restoring the system to complete health. Many can 'lift' melancholy and depression; others are nocturnal and daytime tranquillizers, and there are teas to alleviate pain and clear the skin, also herbal infusions for external uses as poultices and skin-tonics. *Includes:* Carminative teas 'for comforting the stomacke'; Cosmetic teas 'for helping to beautify the skin'; Pain-killing teas 'for allaying the agony'; Febrifuge teas 'to allay the fever'; Teas to induce sleep 'and to help settle obstreporous spirits'.

VITAMINS

WHAT THEY ARE AND WHY WE NEED THEM

Carol Hunter. Explains the characteristics of all known vitamins, their role in health and nutrition, the deficiency symptoms that occur when they are not found in the diet. Includes chapters on improving one's appearance, individual vitamin needs, minimizing vitamin loss in cooking, and megavitamin therapy for alcoholism, schizophrenia, and other diseases. *Other contents:* The discovery of Niacin; E for fertility; Where to find vitamin A; Spotting a deficiency; The role of Thiamine; Why we need vitamin C; Assessing your requirements; Brewer's yeast for B vitamins; The value of wheat germ; Molasses—a nutritious sweetener; Growing your own bean sprouts; Planning your own daily diet.

THE RAW FOOD WAY TO HEALTH

CHANGE YOUR EATING HABITS AND CHANGE YOUR LIFE

Janet Hunt. Raw is healthy! Good health, says the author, is something we all want; and yet our modern life-style with its scientifically produced convenience foods does little to encourage healthy living. But by adopting a raw food diet the body is supplied with all the vitamins, minerals and roughage it needs in a way it can easily assimilate. The author gives a list of delicious salad combinations to show that raw food living need not be a dreary, unimaginative process. Also includes: raw food as a cure for common ailments, home-growing, buying raw food.

ABOUT GINSENG

The Magical Herb of the East

Stephen Fulder, M.A., Ph.D. Ginseng, the strange 'man-shaped' root of the Orient, has been used as a panacea for thousands of years in the East. Now it is freely available in the West, notably from health food stores, and Stephen Fulder explains exactly where and how Ginseng is cultivated; the different forms available; its effect on the ageing process; its value in treating cardiovascular disease, sexual impotence, depression, insomnia, and many other conditions. *Part contents:* Ginseng and herbal medicine in China; Ginseng as stimulant and sedative; Ginseng and potency; What does Ginseng contain?; How to take Ginseng; Ginseng today.

BRAN

HOW BRAN REPLACES FIBRE MISSING FROM TODAY'S DIET, THUS ELIMINATING CONSTIPATION AND COLONIC DISEASES

Ray Hill. Apart from relieving constipation and other bowel disorders, such as colitis and diverticulitis, bran also fulfils an important function in the slimming diet which is both physical and psychological in that it creates in a meal bulk which is not absorbed by the body. This book shows how to use bran in the daily preparation of meals, and there are a number of tasty recipes for bran breads, biscuits, scones and puddings; plus a selection of bran breakfast ideas, bran drinks, and even bran for the skin.

HOW TO EAT FOR HEALTH

DIET REFORM SIMPLIFIED

Stanley Lief N.D. An authority on the question of dietetics, Stanley Lief maintained that the fundamental truths of scientific diet are unchangeable. In this book he has embodied the most important information necessary for those who wish to eat wisely, know when to eat, how much to eat, what to eat, and the most healthful method of preparing their food. All these vital facts are presented by the author in simple, succinct language. Over seventy mouth-watering recipes are included. *Other contents:* The importance of food; Chief dietary faults; Construction of a rational diet; The 'no-breakfast' plan; The question of dessert; Contamination by aluminium.

VEGETARIAN COOKER-TOP COOKERY

DELICIOUS, WHOLESOME, MEAT-FREE MEALS WITHOUT USING AN OVEN

Pamela Brown. For all who live in bed-sitters or who wish to cook on a self-catering holiday, in a caravan, a boat, or outdoors—and for those who don't want to waste fuel by heating a whole oven for just one meal. Packed with essential protein value, these recipes include Bread, Scones and Pancakes; Pasta and Pizzas; Rice and other grains; Eggs, nuts; Salads, sauces, soups and sweets.